# SHOCK THERAPY FOR THE AMERICAN HEALTH CARE SYSTEM

# Shock Therapy for the American Health Care System

## Why Comprehensive Reform Is Needed

*Robert A. Levine, M.D.*

**PRAEGER**

*An Imprint of ABC-CLIO, LLC*

A B C 🛆 C L I O

Santa Barbara, California • Denver, Colorado • Oxford, England

Copyright © 2009 by Robert A. Levine, M.D.

**Library of Congress Cataloging-in-Publication Data**

Cataloging-in-Publication Data is on file with the Library of Congress

ISBN: 978-0-313-38068-6

E-ISBN: 978-0-313-38069-3

13  12  11  10  9    1  2  3  4  5

This book is also available on the World Wide Web as an eBook.
Visit www.abc-clio.com for details.

ABC-CLIO, LLC
130 Cremona Drive, P.O. Box 1911
Santa Barbara, California 93116-1911

This book is printed on acid-free paper ∞
Manufactured in the United States of America

*To Isabel, my granddaughter,*
*whose generation will bear the burdens of*
*our health care profligacy unless corrective measures are taken.*

# CONTENTS

# Contents

# FOREWORD

Dr. Robert Levine is to be greatly complimented for so diligently researching this mammoth, complicated topic crisscrossed with each industry's own agenda and bias. In my opinion, some of Dr. Levine's suggestions for reform are very worthwhile, whereas others need further deliberation. It amuses as well as saddens me that most ideas of health care reform entertained in Congress are built not from the patients' perspective but from the stakeholders' perspective, especially how the reform will bring more turf or revenue to the stakeholder. True health care reform can only happen when our leaders design a plan for the good of the patient first, then wrap around this plan the necessary medical, business, and legal steps to have it implemented. Each stakeholder has to come to the table to give and not to take and hoard. We are all patients at one time or another. "Do unto others what you want others to do unto you."

Again, bravo to Dr. Levine for a gargantuan task well done.

K. J. Lee, M.D., F.A.C.S.
Former vice chair of an HMO insurance
Past chair of a hospital board and medical staff
Past president of national, state, and local medical societies
Associate Clinical Professor, Yale University
Emeritus Chief of Otolaryngology, Hospital of St. Raphael

# ACKNOWLEDGMENTS

Dr. Stephen Levinson was of invaluable assistance in reviewing my manuscript. Offering incisive comments and helpful hints, he brought better focus to some of my ideas and greater coherence to some of my passages.

My wife, Anne, was there as always, critiquing my concepts and use of language, and bringing me down to earth when I was off in the stratosphere. This book would never have been finished without her support, encouragement, and practical advice.

Finally, I would like to thank my editor, Debora Carvalko, who helped bring this project to fruition.

Robert A. Levine, M.D.
April 20, 2009

CHAPTER 1

# INTRODUCTION
## Addressing the Myths about
## Health Care Reform

> The common good is everywhere clearly apparent, and only good sense is needed to perceive it.
>
> —Jean-Jacques Rousseau[1]

The United States needs comprehensive health care reform. Its health care system is broken beyond repair, with annual costs soaring. One-sixth of the population lacks access to care, while those with health insurance find the premiums, co-pays, and deductibles continuously rising, causing care to be less affordable. And in this period of economic turmoil, the absence of secure and reasonable coverage for many Americans makes their finances, as well as their health, even more precarious. But aside from the immediate consequences for individuals and the economy, the unfunded liabilities of Medicare and Medicaid are climbing into the trillions of dollars. These long-term obligations will place a tremendous financial burden on the backs of today's children and succeeding generations, making this country's prosperity more tenuous in the future.

To address this crisis in health care, a number of proposals for reform have been advanced by politicians and economists. When scrutinized, however, these proposals are seen to be halfway measures that are doomed to failure, without realistic cost constraints included in the programs. Like pouring gasoline on a fire, the proposals for the most part employ insurance companies and free market policies to implement reform, strategies that are responsible for the crisis in the first place. Fortunately, the economic problems linked to runaway health care costs are not a foregone conclusion. Comprehensive reform can derail the train of cost acceleration from its tracks and restore rationality to health care expenditures. In fact, though it may be hard to fathom, intelligent reform measures (as will be shown) can not only slow the growth in health care spending, but can reduce costs below levels that have been accepted as normal.

Comprehensive health care reform (CHCR) is what its name implies—a collection of reform measures encompassing all aspects of health care to bring about a complete restructuring of the current system. It would replace the piecemeal, incremental changes that have been introduced periodically since the passage of Medicare over 40 years ago, which have not resolved the major problems, and have in fact made matters worse. The nascent reform plans now being offered fit into the same category and would not end the health care crisis. But relief can occur if U.S. politicians leave behind their parochial concerns and think in grand terms, realizing that comprehensive reform is the only solution. It will take a concerted effort by the president and the Congress to pass the necessary legislation. This endeavor must involve negotiation and compromise by both political parties, and must place practicality and common sense above ideology. Given the plight of the health care system, new vision and creative action are required from the nation's elected officials—qualities that have not often been in evidence.

Nearly a century has passed since Teddy Roosevelt first raised the possibility of national health insurance for Americans, with a number of unsuccessful efforts to enact programs since that time. In addition to proposals by Teddy and later Franklin Roosevelt, national health insurance was again suggested by President Harry Truman after World War II in 1945, with 75 percent of the population supporting the idea.[2] (By 1949, however only 21 percent were in favor, having been convinced by those opposed that the concept was communist-inspired.) Only Medicare legislation for the elderly and disabled in the 1960s and Medicaid were able to overcome the powerful forces arrayed against reform, including organized medicine and the pharmaceutical and health insurance industries. Though universal coverage has never gotten off the ground, with the recent astronomical rise in health care costs, and with employers, workers, and other consumers crying out for relief, the time is ripe for another try. The current general economic dislocation makes this even more imperative.

Health care reform was one of the three top issues of the 2008 presidential campaign, with plans formulated by the contenders in both parties as templates for change. The desire for change by citizens is not new. A survey as far back as 1984 revealed that 51 percent of Americans favored extensive modifications of health care delivery and 31 percent believed a complete overhaul was necessary.[3] Current advocates for change invariably use the structures in place as the basis for reform, including government options and private insurance companies to provide health insurance coverage. These plans, shaped by political considerations, will not correct existing problems. And if incomplete or unsatisfactory reform measures are enacted, they may be the law of the land for years, putting further pressure on the economy and society. America must have comprehensive reform that will provide access to care for everyone, rein in runaway costs, and simplify the entire system. The nation cannot afford to wait much longer.

I am a physician who has been in private practice (neurology) for over 35 years. During this period, I have dealt with the obstacles and inconsistencies of the health care system and the insurance labyrinth on a daily basis. My office has tried to assist legions of patients who were attempting to navigate their way to reimbursement or approval for various tests and treatments in a Kafkaesque arrangement designed to make it difficult for people to find answers to simple questions. These include young and old, wealthy and poor, sophisticated and naïve—all frustrated by the insurance barriers placed in their way. I have also seen how the health care system has evolved over the last several decades, adding to its complexity and increasing its cost, without a corresponding improvement in care. I bring a different perspective to the need for health care reform than do the multitude of politicians, economists, and academics who have proposed remedies for this burgeoning crisis.

If this nation's dysfunctional health care system is to undergo the kind of transformation that will allow it to provide first-rate care to its citizens in a cost-effective manner, it is essential that certain myths about it be dispelled. Over the years, these fables have been promulgated by special interest groups and political ideologues who are opposed to reform. They would like to either maintain the status quo or shape the changes that may be in store, maximizing the benefits they will receive. Among the myths that need to be repudiated, eight stand out, some believed overwhelmingly by most Americans, others accepted by large segments of the population. It is important that the politicians and the public recognize these myths to give the former a greater chance of getting it right when health care reform comes up before Congress, and to help the latter understand why the process has been so difficult.

*Myth #1: Americans have the best health care in the world.* A number of statistics belie that claim, showing that the United States actually ranks near the bottom on several standard criteria.[4] Although a small percentage of the most affluent may be able to obtain excellent medical intervention, the United States places only 42nd among all nations in life expectancy according to data from the Census Bureau and the National Center for Health Statistics.[5] (Twenty years earlier, the United States ranked 11th.) Most European citizens, the Japanese, and the Jordanians, among others, live longer than Americans. And among industrialized nations, the United States now ranks last in preventable mortality.[6] Another important objective metric, infant mortality, has the United States at 41st, with most of Europe, Cuba, and Taiwan having better survival rates.[7] As disheartening as these numbers may be, there is yet another important statistic that argues against the quality of this country's health care: almost 46 million people are uninsured and unable to obtain reliable medical services; about one-sixth of America's population.[8] In the developed world, America alone does not provide medical care for all of its citizens. A report to Congress last year comparing the quality of care in the United States against that of other industrialized nations also found America lagging, even if the uninsured were not considered. There were only 2.4 practicing physicians per 1,000 population, which placed the United States in the bottom third of affluent countries.[9] It was also more difficult to get same-day appointments than elsewhere, and care was often suboptimal on nights and weekends.

Obtaining care is a problem not only for the uninsured, but also for those who might be considered "underinsured." These are individuals and families who have health insurance but cannot afford the high deductibles or co-pays, or whose policies don't cover the tests or treatments they require. As the cost of health care has skyrocketed, companies that provide insurance for their employees have sought to control expenses by opting for less inclusive plans, which means more out-of-pocket costs for those needing medical assistance. In a struggling economy, it is even more difficult for many people to come up with those extra dollars. A survey revealed that 20 percent of Americans, about 59 million people, either delayed or did not go for necessary care in 2003, when the economy was stronger, because of a lack of insurance or inadequate coverage.[10] This is certainly even more of a problem since the onset of the financial meltdown. Those on Medicaid also have trouble obtaining appropriate care, as many physicians won't see these patients because of insufficient reimbursement.

*Myth #2: Private insurance companies deliver care that is less expensive and more efficient than does the government.* Notwithstanding this oft-repeated mantra by politicians and health insurance companies, government-run health care programs in the United States consistently perform better and are more economical than private insurance-based plans. Medicare, the government program for people over 65 and the disabled, is less complex and less costly than the insurance plans created by for-profit companies. It is less confusing for patients and has fewer rules for physicians, eliminating preauthorization for most tests and treatments. With reduced administrative and overhead expenditures compared to private insurance, more of its funds can be devoted to patient care. Similarly, the Veterans Administration (VA) system run by the government offers less costly, more efficient care than the private sector. VA hospitals have scored considerably higher than private institutions on the University of Michigan's American Customer Satisfaction Index for a number of years, and their death rate is 40 percent lower for men over 65 than for those in private Medicare plans.[11]

Interestingly, to support private Medicare Advantage plans, which Republicans had been pushing, the Bush administration was willing to pay participating insurance companies an extra premium above and beyond the regular Medicare costs, because Medicare Advantage could not provide care for older patients as inexpensively.[12] These private plans received an average of 13–17 percent more from the government to furnish the same services as traditional Medicare.[13] It has been estimated that the government will pay an extra $50 billion to the insurance companies running the private plans from

2009 to 2012 for these subsidies. This further debunks the notion that private companies can deliver medical care more efficiently and less expensively than the government. (Because these plans are profitable with the extra payments they receive, insurance companies have been aggressively trying to persuade older people to sign up and drop regular Medicare, using misleading claims about benefits and other deceptive practices to convince them to change.[14] Agents have been paid commissions of up to $600 for every person they enroll.)

*Myth #3: Health care reform is bound to lower quality and result in inferior care for those patients who already have insurance coverage, while increasing their costs.* Statistics show that Americans' health care is currently in need of improvement across the board, and the proper reforms should make things better rather than worse. In addition to raising quality through more oversight and quality control innovations, costs per patient are likely to go down as more people are covered, particularly if the hordes of young, healthy men and women who are now without insurance are brought into the system. (Though costs per patient will diminish, if 46 million Americans are suddenly covered by health insurance, it is inevitable that overall expenditures will rise unless measures to constrain costs are instituted. Although many of the uninsured are healthy, there are large numbers with chronic illnesses who have not received care previously. When coverage is available for them, they will go to physicians' offices seeking help, generating more diagnostic tests and more treatments for their ailments, indeed, more services of every sort.)

*Myth #4: Expensive care, the kind many Americans receive, is synonymous with better care.* Considerably more money is spent per capita for health care in the United States than in any other country,[15] yet the results are poor, as has been shown. (The United States spent $6,401 for each person in 2005, compared to Norway at $4,364 and Switzerland at $4,177, the next highest countries.[16]) Actually, expensive care for symptoms and illnesses is often the result of excessive tests and treatments that may be medically unnecessary. And some of these procedures can cause injuries or adverse outcomes that would not have otherwise occurred, negatively affecting patients' health in addition to increasing costs. Preventive medicine, watchful waiting and conservative therapy for various conditions often produces better results for patients at lower cost than expensive, aggressive treatments. The Center for Evaluative Clinical Sciences at Dartmouth Medical school has estimated that "20 to 30 percent of health care spending goes for procedures, office visits, drugs, hospitalizations, and treatments that do absolutely nothing to improve the quality or increase the length of our lives—but which nonetheless drive up costs. At the same time, the type of treatment that offers clear benefits is not reaching many Americans, even those who are insured."[17] Evidence is given to bolster these assertions showing that "the supply of medical services rather than the demand for them determines the amount of care given."[18, 19]

*Myth #5: America's health care system has been carefully planned and well thought out, the product of constructive political dialogue over the years.*

***Thus, it should merely be tweaked slightly to improve its efficiency and func-
tioning.*** In fact, the current structure evolved haphazardly from its inception
during World War II. With government wage controls in place at that time,
companies decided to offer health insurance to help them recruit new personnel.
(This approach has regrettably linked coverage to employment for working-age
men and women ever since.) Physicians and other providers set their own
charges and were reimbursed on a fee-for-service basis by the insurance companies. In 1965, Medicare was enacted to provide health care to seniors and the
disabled, along with Medicaid for those who were impoverished. Subsequently,
managed care arrived in force in the 1990s with its multiple permutations
(HMOs, PPOs, etc.) in an attempt to control exploding costs. Though the rate
of increase was dampened for a short period as approvals for services and reimbursement were cut, it soon resumed its upward flight. (Health care spending
rose three to five times the growth in overall wages and prices from 2001 to
2005 according to the National Coalition on Health Care.[20]) The latest additions
to the stew—an attempt to help individuals pay for care—are Health Savings
Accounts (HSAs), which do nothing to solve the basic problems.

Unfortunately, the chaotic development of America's health care system, with
its mix of private and government programs, has resulted in a smorgasbord of
great complexity that prevents citizens from understanding the choices available to them. Every private insurance company has a number of individual plans,
each with a different array of costs, coverages, co-pays, deductibles, need for preauthorization, and the like. This complexity makes it all but impossible for even
the most sophisticated consumers to be able to decipher their options. It also
makes it challenging for physicians to provide the care their patients need.

***Myth #6: There is no health care crisis, merely a few kinks in the system
that will respond to minor adjustments.*** In fact, aside from the nearly 46 million people without coverage and the poor quality of care, prohibitive costs negatively impact those who do have insurance, companies that offer it to their
employees, the federal and state governments, and the entire U.S. economy. The
nation's corporations have had difficulty managing their health care costs for
decades, with a number of companies dropping their plans, others choosing less
comprehensive coverage, and others shifting more of the expense to their
employees. Spending on health care also makes American products less competitive worldwide, with legacy costs—health care plus pensions—for U.S.
automakers estimated at about $1,500 or more per vehicle.[21] In addition, when
businesses pay more for health insurance for their employees, they recoup some
of the costs by paying their employees less, resulting in diminished spending
power and a lower standard of living for those workers. The rise in health care
costs also comes out of Americans' pockets in the form of increased state and
federal taxes to support the Medicare and Medicaid programs. Spending for
health care currently accounts for the single largest portion of state budgets.[22]

As mentioned above, some people with insurance cannot afford their components of care and may avoid doctors' visits, delay tests or omit required

medications. (Health care expenses are a major cause of personal bankruptcy.) Sixteen percent of the American economy is now devoted to health care ($2.1 trillion[23]) with estimates that this will rise to 20 percent by 2015 ($4 trillion) and may go even higher with further aging of the population.[24] There are some economists who say that as a rich country we can afford to spend a large proportion of our wealth on health care.[25] But this is money that cannot be utilized in other areas, such as education, research, homeland security, the military, and paying down the national debt. The United States spends 4.3 times more on health care than on national defense.[26] Comparable percentages of GDP spent on health care are 10.7 percent for Germany, 9.7 percent for Canada and 9.5 percent for France.[27] Yet the extraordinary expenditures by the United States fail to provide first-rate care for its citizens.

With the government's portion of the nation's medical bill (paid through Medicare, Medicaid, and the VA system) growing rapidly, estimates of future unfunded liabilities for health care are believed to be in the trillions to tens of trillions of dollars. While Social Security costs rose only 5 percent from 2000 to 2007, Medicare costs increased 55 percent.[28] A report by the Bush administration in March 2008 noted that Medicare's hospital insurance trust fund would be depleted by 2019.[29] Thus far, elected officials have been unwilling to address these elements of the health care crisis along with the other aspects that have been described. The longer cost constraints and funding of these obligations are not a priority, the harder it will be to devise solutions, and the more pain America's citizens will ultimately suffer. Worried about the reaction from their constituents, politicians avoid even speaking about the problem or trying to educate the electorate about it. Better to leave it for the next generation.

*Myth #7: Comprehensive health care reform is unaffordable in these tough economic times, bound to increase taxes as well as America's budget deficit and national debt.* This may be true of the major plans currently on the table, all of which lack credible cost constraints, but a comprehensive program that is carefully constructed could potentially save the government (and individuals) vast amounts of money, make the nation's businesses more competitive, and spur economic growth, even as it improves the quality of care. There are huge savings waiting to be harvested in America's bloated health care system with a program that aggressively attacks and reduces administrative costs, fraud, and unnecessary care. However, extensive changes will be required in the way health care is paid for and delivered—changes that will be opposed by organized medicine, hospitals, and the health insurance and pharmaceutical industries, all of whom will have to surrender some of the special benefits and advantages they now perceive as their birthright.

*Myth #8 (which is trumpeted loudly by politicians from both parties as well as the concerned special interests): Free market policies are the desired way to solve the dilemmas of the health care system.* This idea is misguided at best, since the market usually performs poorly when applied to health care. An article in the *Journal of the American Medical Association* in 2007 explained why the free market is inefficient in terms of health care, noting that there was imperfect competition, with a market where an individual buyer or seller could influence the price of a service by his or her actions.[30] Because of this, market distortions occurred, among which were "asymmetry of information between clinicians and patients; clinicians' dual roles as patient agent and independent business owner (profiting by ordering or providing certain medical services); the effect of insurance in reducing the apparent cost of health care services to patients; . . . tax subsidies that have a similar effect on consumers' decisions to purchase insurance; and monopoly power bestowed on certain professions . . . limiting competition." Unfortunately, American belief in the market as the answer to all economic problems (which many accept on faith) often obscures the reality of some situations, making solutions more difficult.

One example of how people disregard the market in the realm of health care is the way they choose specialists or treatments for critical illnesses. Very few, if any, select the cheapest cardiac surgeon to repair their leaking heart valves, or the low-priced neurosurgeon to operate on their brain tumors, or the least expensive oncologist to treat their cancers. The vast majority want the best doctors when their lives or health are on the line. Similarly, in deciding on therapy, they don't embrace the most economical approach to attack their cancers or other life-threatening medical conditions. They want the ones that will work the best and have the fewest side effects. Of course, it may be difficult for people of limited means who cannot afford medical care to follow this dictum. They may accept whatever options are offered to them. But even in those circumstances, there are some who are willing to go deeply into debt and eventual bankruptcy to get the best care for themselves or their loved ones. The market is certainly not the controlling force in the treatment of serious afflictions.

When individuals "shop" for medical insurance, the market can play a role, but cost is only one of several factors that is taken into account. It is least important for those who are affluent and have the most freedom to make choices, and a more significant consideration for those with lower incomes. In addition to price, most consumers seeking health care coverage use quality as an important determinant and are only satisfied if they believe the best doctors (particularly their own physicians) and the best medical centers are covered in their plans. Businesses, of course, may assess things differently in purchasing group coverage for their workers. Cost usually decides which insurance plans the companies select, though quality and coverage are elements in their equations. However, the main objective for corporations is ostensibly profit for their stockholders (and compensation for their top executives), not the well-being of their employees. When executives are given the opportunity to choose their own insurance plans, they usually pick the best ones available rather than the least expensive.

Another simplified illustration of the way market forces are flouted in health care is the way specialists set their fees to generate income. For instance, in a particular community, general surgeon A earns $300,000 annually performing 300 operations and charging $1,000 for each procedure. Suddenly, a new surgeon, B, enters the community and starts a practice. They both are considered competent, and together they now do 400 operations a year. By market theory, one would expect the two surgeons in competition to reduce their prices in an attempt to attract more patients. However, the opposite usually occurs. When surgeon A discovers his patient load has slipped and he is doing only 200 operations each year, he still wants to maintain his standard of living and earn $300,000 annually. So instead of dropping his fees, he increases them, now charging $1,500 for each procedure. His competitor, surgeon B, who would also like a high standard of living, charges $1,500 as well, with market forces not limiting the price increases. (They do not collude to set their fees, arriving at their charges independently, so they are not breaking antitrust laws.)

Perhaps the two surgeons find, however, that there are only 350 operations required by the community each year and they are reluctant to raise their prices higher than $1,500 per procedure. Then one or both physicians may decide to change the criteria he or she employs to determine a patient's need for surgery, lowering the bar and operating in questionable situations. By taking this step, they will be able to earn more money by performing more operations. Of course, this action also distorts the market, with physicians creating unnecessary work in order to maintain their incomes. This scenario happens not infrequently in U.S. medicine, where there is often a conflict of interest between a physician's economic gain and good patient care.

Insurance companies and Medicare currently act as constraining forces on the fees charged (also distorting the market) for those medical practitioners who are participants. These entities set the reimbursement rates for all medical procedures and treatments involving the patients they cover, not allowing participating physicians to raise their charges unilaterally. Though physicians can opt out of these programs in order to establish their own fees, only a minority choose to do so, as it means they will be excluded from third-party reimbursement. (If physicians are nonparticipants, money from third-party payers may go directly to the patients themselves, who do not always use it to pay their doctors.) Insurance companies and Medicare are also supposed to monitor physicians to try and prevent unnecessary procedures. But accurate monitoring is not easily accomplished, and many physicians do in fact increase their volume of work with superfluous procedures to produce more income.

Another element working against the market is the fact that no physician wants to be known as the cheap provider in a community. Many people still equate price with quality in medical care and are reluctant to choose physicians who are regarded as inexpensive. Patients (as well as some physicians) believe that a doctor who does not value his or her services highly must not be as good as one who charges more. This belief also works against competition based on price. Perhaps if there were correlative stratification between fees charged and the quality of services, one could say that the market might be playing a role and that it made sense to pay more for a superior product in terms of medical care. Unfortunately, there is no correlation between the two elements and no accurate metric to help consumers (patients) make decisions about whether to spend more for a particular physician's service.

Although there are available statistics regarding surgeons' operative mortality and morbidity, these do not inform the layman about the relative difficulty of the cases undertaken by each surgeon. For instance, a highly skilled surgeon might operate on patients who are sicker and at greater risk, while a more pedestrian one would avoid them. The former might thus have a lower statistical profile even though he or she was more proficient than his or her colleague. And measuring the competence of the majority of physicians who do not perform operations is even more daunting, as there are few parameters to guide the consumer's choice of doctor. The magazines who pronounce "the best doctors" in a community are often off-base in their assessments and list only a small proportion of all physicians. Insurance company ratings are linked more to price than to quality, as an investigation by the New York attorney general in 2007 corroborated.[31] And online rating sites are rarely employed by patients to make decisions about care and may be inaccurate.[32]

Because of the lack of available objective information, there are several ways patients pick their physicians, or decide to stay with the ones they have chosen. The first (and most important) factor is affability, or so-called "bedside manner," which has nothing to do with competence. If patients believe a doctor is compassionate, understands their needs, and communicates well with them, they are satisfied and want to use that doctor for their care. (This is usually independent of cost, but not always. If there is not a long-standing relationship, patients may seek new physicians if their insurance coverage changes and does not include their old doctors.) Convenience and availability are also factors when people select primary care physicians. The second way people find or keep physicians is through word-of-mouth—recommendations by friends or family members. If friends declare that a doctor is good, a person will feel comfortable and tend to use him or her. However, friends generally also use affability, which they confuse with ability, as their criterion when they endorse a doctor. The third way physicians are selected is through referrals from other physicians. While competence is more likely a consideration here, referrals may be directed by a physician to his or her friends, or someone who will refer back. Local hospitals or insurance plans are also used as a source for physician referrals. In all of these situations, a patient's choice of physician is not determined by the market.

An article in the *New England Journal of Medicine* in 1999 noted that "an informed choice by consumers, which results in efficiency according to market theory, is a mirage in health care. Many patients (e.g., frail elderly patients and those who are seriously ill, who account for the largest proportion of hospital care) cannot comparison shop, reduce their demand for services when suppliers raise prices, or accurately appraise quality."[33]

The geographical maldistribution of physicians in America is another illustration of the inability of the market to solve health care problems. Physicians entering practice do not necessarily gravitate to the places where they can make the most money (or where they are needed the most). Many tend to cluster in urban areas (those that are not economically depressed or largely minority), where there is a high ratio of doctors to the population, often neglecting mid-size and smaller towns where additional physicians may be in greater demand. The surfeit of physicians in some cities may make it more difficult to start practices there and generate high incomes, and the cost of living is usually greater. This may be rectified by doctors working longer hours and charging higher fees for services. The appeal of large cities to physicians is not financial. Instead, they are influenced by the availability of cultural activities, the quality of life, intellectual stimulation, better hospital facilities, the proximity of other physicians, and so forth.

According to market theory, when hospitals compete in the same or adjacent communities for specialized services, costs for those services should decrease. However, when hospitals vie for the same population of patients, they do not generally do so by reducing fees. Instead, they emphasize the quality of the services offered or the physicians involved, convenience, or nonmedical incentives. The quest for status between neighboring institutions often leads them to buy the same or similar expensive equipment and target the same fixed pool of patients for particular services (instead of cooperating on the purchase and sharing the equipment, or having one institution specialize in one medical sphere and a neighboring institution in a different one). This often results in the hospitals' providing the service at a loss or at a break-even level, even though the fees are high. Having the most modern equipment and being able to perform complex diagnostic tests and innovative procedures may be a point of pride for the hospitals and is seen by their leaders as building prestige. But it does not make economic sense. In fact, it may not even make sense medically. It has been shown that the success rate for many difficult medical procedures is directly related to the number performed at an institution and that complications rise inversely to that number. Concentrating the procedures at fewer institutions would lead to better outcomes.

Hospitals are also legally required to provide services to patients, whether or not they can pay for them, in disregard of the market. This is a reminder that by law and from an ethical standpoint, health care is different than other businesses. Sick patients must be cared for, independent of an assumed financial contract. This places a tremendous burden on institutions where a large percentage of their population base is uninsured. Knowing that hospitals will provide care if something unforeseen happens also serves as an impetus for people to avoid purchasing health insurance. The uninsured realize they will always be able to obtain emergency care and are willing to gamble that they will not become injured or sick, thus saving the money they would spend on insurance. This unfortunately raises costs for those who have insurance, as they wind up subsidizing those who don't. (Hospitals increase their fees for those who can pay to help cover uncompensated services.)

Many hospitals also hold a virtual monopoly in the areas they serve.[34] About 50 percent of Americans reside in communities where the population is too sparse to support medical competition among hospitals or specialists. Unless people living in these areas are willing to travel long distances to receive care, which is often not possible in emergency situations or for economic or logistical reasons, they are forced to use the local institutions and providers, with the market playing no role in their decisions.

For some time now, insurance companies have been attempting to use market incentives to control costs, having failed with other mechanisms. To make their policyholders conscious of costs, they have had them pay a portion of provider's fees through deductibles and co-pays for whatever services are utilized. The hope is that this outlay will induce policyholders to reduce the amount of medical services. However, this strategy does not impact the affluent, and to be truly effective with the middle class, deductibles and co-pays would have to be much higher. Unfortunately, these negative market incentives work mainly as a constraint on the poor who do not see physicians regularly, are often late in seeking treatment for acute problems, and neglect care for chronic conditions. This leads to the worsening of many illnesses and may make patients more refractory to therapy, which ultimately raises health care costs both for individuals and for society.

Of all the health care myths that are accepted as common wisdom by many U.S. politicians and citizens, the biggest impediment to effective reform appears to be the belief that market forces are the best therapy for the current crisis. This is not to say that measures employing the market should be ignored in any reform proposal. However, they must not be the mainstay of any corrective efforts that are put forth. Both political parties (or at least the president and a majority of the legislators in Washington) have to understand that the market is not the solution to the problems of health care. This will mean overcoming strongly held convictions that are constantly reinforced by the political and economic rhetoric of free-marketeers. These individuals and groups label any expansion of government involvement in health care as "socialized medicine" and refuse to recognize the success of the Medicare program, which has been a boon to America's elderly for over 40 years. Through subsidies and direct payments, the government already pays for over 60 percent of the country's health care expenditures, as has been noted by some economists.[35] U.S. government spending on health care was shown to equal 9.6 percent of GDP in 2004, compared to 6.9 percent in Canada, which has a single-payer, universal health care system. In the current arrangement, with so much waste and redundancy, the United States is certainly not getting enough bang for its buck.

Of course, some of these same free-marketeers have recently been willing to support a federal bailout of the troubled investment banking system, the takeover of Fannie Mae and Freddie Mac, the rescue of the AIG insurance company, and loans to the auto industry, rather than allowing the market to hold sway in those instances. Deregulation of the market for electricity, using free market principles, has been a disaster, with electricity prices for consumers ballooning in states with competitive pricing compared to regulated states[36] and windfall profits for some of the energy companies. Indeed, there has been a push in some states for re-regulation of the industry. Similarly, there are many who believe that deregulation of the airline industry was a failure even before the surge in fuel prices occurred, with many companies going bankrupt, loss of jobs, and poor quality of services.

Free-market policies and unfettered capitalism are not always the answer to complex problems. The market encourages people to do whatever is necessary to make money, and where health care is concerned, that is synonymous with runaway costs and poor quality of care. The Nobel Laureate economist Paul Krugman has noted that the United States "has the most privatized system, with the most market competition—and it also has by far the highest health care costs in the world."[37]

There are many who believe that far-reaching changes in this country's health care system should not be considered in the near future given the nation's current economic downturn. However, looking to the past, the most expansive social legislation in American history, Social Security, was enacted during the Great Depression in the 1930s, when the naysayers were overruled. The state of the economy should not stop comprehensive health care reform from being passed, for if it is properly crafted, it will actually save the government money while providing universal access to care.

Whatever plan is ultimately chosen to reconfigure American health care, three elements must be included if it is to be successful.

1. There must be universal (or near-universal) access to care.
2. There must be strong, built-in cost constraints.
3. There must be simplification.

Keeping the myths in mind may lead to more realistic suggestions about how to reform a dysfunctional health care system.

The various options for reform will be discussed in later chapters.

## CHAPTER 2

# EVOLUTION OF THE AMERICAN HEALTH CARE SYSTEM

## The Changing Physician, Organized Medicine, and Efforts at Health Care Reform

> In the human body, when the usual symptoms of health or sickness disappoint our expectation; when medicines operate not with their wonted powers; when irregular events follow from any particular cause; the philosopher and physician are not surprised at the matter.... They know that a human body is a mighty complicated machine: That many secret powers lurk in it, which are altogether beyond our comprehension.
>
> —David Hume, *Enquiries Concerning Human Understanding*[1]

## The Changing Physician

From medieval times through the late nineteenth century, medical practitioners in Western societies were generally regarded by the populace as quacks or parasites who capitalized on the misfortunes of the sick and the dying. With little understanding of the physiology of the human body or the origins of illness, physicians combined the occult and the mystical with occasional dashes of common sense as they ministered to the afflicted, their diagnostic and therapeutic methods generating fear and doubt in their charges. Early physicians commonly believed that disease was caused by an imbalance of four bodily humors that represented different physical elements: blood (air), phlegm (water), black bile (earth), and yellow bile (fire). Treatment consisted of trying to restore the balance of these humors by the removal—through purging—of whichever one they thought was in excess. This meant bleeding patients or using leeches, various emetics, enemas, and blistering plasters administered to individuals who might already be quite ill. Since the afflicted frequently seemed to be injured by the remedies prescribed, physicians were often called to tend the sick as a last resort, further insuring poor outcomes.

Physicians' low status in the eyes of the public was reinforced by the lack of specific requirements or standard courses of study for doctors, as well as the fact that anyone could practice medicine, unrestrained by licensing. Men became doctors by apprenticing themselves to older practitioners or by merely bestowing the title upon themselves, since there were initially no universities or medical schools to provide legitimacy to the profession through diplomas or other credentials. Though the first U.S. medical school was created at the University of Pennsylvania in 1765, followed by Harvard in 1783,[2] these institutions were unusual in teaching a medical curriculum. In addition, physicians did not have hospitals where they could bring their sick patients to recover from serious illnesses. Many had trouble making a living from their practices and some worked at medicine part time, with second jobs to sustain them.

Most Americans in the eighteenth and nineteenth centuries believed in the innate ability of the common man to deal with matters of health in a rational fashion, calling upon the elders of the community for assistance, with self-treatment for most conditions being the accepted norm. Home medical manuals, describing symptoms and illnesses along with the appropriate therapies, were found in nearly all households, particularly in rural areas where doctors were not readily available. These manuals were considered invaluable, dispensing advice to the layman on how to manage various disorders. Folk remedies were also frequently employed.

Another challenge to the status of physicians and their ability to generate income was the large number of practitioners with diverse approaches to illness who called themselves doctors. All claimed that theirs was the best way to care for afflicted patients, while denigrating other schools of thought. The competing orders included botanic medicine, whose most prominent advocate was Samuel Thomson, eclectic medicine, which combined several approaches, and homeopathy which was in vogue from the early to mid-nineteenth century. Homeopaths believed that for drugs to be effective they should induce symptoms in healthy individuals similar to the diseases they were expected to treat. The drugs would be greatly diluted, then given to patients in small doses and built up gradually in the hope of inducing a response.

Osteopathy was another alternative method of medical treatment, whose tenets were conceived by a physician, Andrew Still, in the 1870s.[3] Osteopaths considered the body to be a machine that could be fixed by manipulation of its parts, to help the circulation and correct altered mechanics. The first osteopathic medical school was founded in Kirksville, Missouri, in 1892, with others following. Eventually, these schools adopted curriculums similar to those of the allopathic (traditional) medical schools. The two types of practices became virtually indistinguishable in the last half of the twentieth century, with shared internships, residencies, and licensing exams.

Chiropractic medicine was started by a magnetic healer, D. D. Palmer, in Davenport, Iowa in 1891.[4] This approach promoted spinal manipulation as a cure for medical problems, while staking its own claim to the medical dollar. In many ways it was similar to osteopathy, though it asserted a different mechanism of action (reducing heat from the friction of misaligned parts). Although osteopathy embraced the ideas and treatments of traditional medicine over time, chiropractors diverged further and continued to employ spinal manipulation to treat illness, despite the lack of scientific evidence that it was beneficial.

Others who advertised themselves as doctors, such as the dispensers of patent medicines, also competed with traditional physicians in the latter half of the nineteenth and early twentieth centuries. With their quack cures, which were embraced by gullible (and not-so-gullible) citizens, they tarnished the image of all medical practitioners. Itinerant peddlers would often make the rounds of rural towns in their mobile clinics (painted wagons), hawking miracle potions for everything from lumbago to senility. There was no vetting of their claims by scientific journals or government agencies, and patients would attest to the effects of these concoctions that were usually fortified with alcohol, cocaine, or opium, either alone or in combination. Some of these "medications" were also sold through newspaper ads and were available by mail order. When the U.S. Food and Drug Administration (FDA) was created in the 1920s and proof was required for assertions of effectiveness, most of the patent medicine makers were forced out of business, though some successor products remain on pharmacy shelves with vague claims of curative powers.

Naturopaths joined the mix of alternative practitioners in the early twentieth century, advocating "natural treatments" that included diet, hygiene, hydrotherapy, spine manipulation, and the use of herbal medicines to treat illnesses.

Allopathic medicine was not static during this period of intense competition with other types of practitioners, but drew on scientific advances and new knowledge to attain a preeminent position with the public in the diagnosis and treatment of illness. One of the major underpinnings of its emergence from the crowded field of medical pretenders was the germ theory of disease, which originated in the mid-nineteenth century, leading to a better understanding of the causes of infectious diseases. Ignaz Semmelweis, a Hungarian obstetrician, in 1847 deduced that puerperal (childbirth) fever was a contagious disease involving unseen organisms.[5] He had all physicians at his hospital wash their hands with water and lime prior to the deliveries, which cut the death rate from 30 percent to less than 2 percent, though the medical establishment was still unconvinced of the validity of his theory. (Today, hospitals are again reducing recently increased rates of infection by requiring all personnel to wash their hands before each patient encounter.)

Further work by John Snow during the 1854 London cholera epidemic, and Louis Pasteur's studies on the growth of micro-organisms in nutrient broth, reinforced the germ theory of disease. Robert Koch in the 1870s validated the concept in the minds of medical scientists and the educated public when he proved that anthrax was transmitted by bacteria. His demonstration technique, known as Koch's postulates, is still employed today to uncover the micro-organisms causing new infections.

Another discovery that helped to power allopathic medicine to the forefront of the medical marketplace was the discovery of anesthesia and its use in surgery. Nitrous oxide (laughing gas) was used by the British chemist Humphrey Davy in 1795, but not utilized in dentistry until 1844.[6] In 1842 Crawford Williamson Long employed chemical anesthesia (diethyl ether) for the first time in a surgical procedure. By 1847 chloroform had replaced ether as the anesthetic of choice as it was less dangerous and had fewer side effects. Over time, newer agents were developed that were even easier to manage. As the use of general anesthesia spread, new therapeutic avenues opened up for patients and physicians. With pain no longer an impediment, people were willing to undergo arduous surgical procedures they had previously rejected. Appendicitis, bleeding ulcers, and inflamed gall bladders could all be managed with relatively simple operations that could be life saving. Amputations could be performed and severe fractures set appropriately without causing unbearable pain. More complicated cancer surgery involving different organs also became possible. Anesthesia not only made surgery a practical choice for patients, but aided the surgeons as well, as their subjects were no longer moving, writhing, and screaming on the operating tables. Physicians and surgeons were now perceived by the public as offering real therapeutic options for treating diseases.

Twenty years after anesthesia was first employed, antiseptic surgical techniques were introduced by the British surgeon Joseph Lister—a major medical advance that cut the risk of perioperative infections. In operations Lister performed at Kings Hospital in London in 1867, he used phenol (carbolic acid) as an antiseptic agent, which dramatically reduced the rate of infection in his patients and revolutionized the practice of surgery worldwide.[7] Further modifications included the sterilization of instruments, careful hand washing, and the use of rubber gloves, caps, and gowns. Robert Koch initiated steam cleaning of surgical instruments to eliminate bacteria, which eventually resulted in sterilization of all materials used in the operating room (OR) to produce aseptic (free from infectious material) surgical fields.

William Stewart Halstead, a towering figure in U.S. surgery, inaugurated and popularized a host of important ideas and techniques during his tenure as chief of surgery at Johns Hopkins Hospital in Baltimore during the late nineteenth and early twentieth century.[8] As these were disseminated throughout the country, they changed the way surgery was performed in the United States. In addition to complete sterility in the operating room and hemostasis of the surgical site (control of bleeding), he originated the use of surgical gloves, gentle handling of tissues, and proper wound closure with alignment of the tissues. Halstead was also responsible for the creation of the first surgical residency program in the

United States, with his acolytes carrying his messages to other hospitals after their training was completed.

The next important development came from Wilhelm Roentgen in 1895. While working with vacuum tubes, he found that x-ray pictures were able to show the body's bone structure, as well as some of the internal tissues.[9] This was a transformational discovery for physicians, enabling them to diagnose the extent of traumatic injuries, fractures of all sorts, pneumonia, lung tumors, and other abnormalities. Initially, most of the new x-ray machines were owned by businessmen who offered curious members of the public "Roentgen photographs" of their bones.[10] During the early years of the new century, physicians sent their patients to these commercial ventures to obtain the x-rays they thought were necessary. However, during the next decade, more hospitals acquired x-ray equipment and some physicians purchased their own machines. A number of doctors even began specializing in a new field called radiology, focusing on x-ray diagnosis.

Other discoveries also elevated medical science and the standing of traditional physicians during the late nineteenth and early twentieth century, though none were as earthshaking as those already described. Still, the utilization of electrocardiography in the diagnosis of heart attacks and cardiac arrhythmias in the second and third decades of the twentieth century was a significant breakthrough. The use of blood transfusions to treat blood loss and shock was also a major development. However, it was not until blood banks were established during and after World War I that blood could be stored and transfusions became a viable option in many situations.

Though the above scientific discoveries were important for allopathic physicians and their patients, questions remained about the quality of medical schools and physicians' training, along with licensing to show that physicians were qualified. Though more medical schools were founded that incorporated the new scientific discoveries into their curricula, there was still not a standard course of study that had to be covered in all institutions. In addition, the admission criteria for medical schools did not always yield high-caliber students. Two events changed medical education and further enhanced the standing of allopathic physicians. The first was increasingly stringent licensing exams for physicians by the states. The second was the Flexner report on medical education that was released in 1910.

The Flexner report is considered the defining event in U.S. medical education in the twentieth century. Abraham Flexner was an educator, not a physician, who worked for the Carnegie Foundation. In his research on the status of medical education and training, he investigated all of the nation's 155 medical schools. His report concluded that standards in these schools varied greatly, with numerous proprietary institutions more interested in turning a profit than in turning out skilled and knowledgeable physicians. The facilities and teachers in some of the schools were mediocre or worse, though others affiliated with universities, such as Johns Hopkins, were excellent.[11] Flexner suggested that U.S. medical schools should follow the German model of teaching the biomedical sciences, along with hands on clinical training, integrating patient care, teaching, and research. Many schools closed after the report was issued, with the rest adopting Flexner's ideas for reform. The basic medical sciences such as anatomy, physiology, and pathology were taught in the first two years of medical school, with clinical apprenticeships and hospital training in years three and four. The new graduates from these schools were better prepared to manage patients and illness, and the prestige and stature of these doctors grew significantly.

Though there were attempts at medical licensing in some of the colonies and states in the eighteenth and early nineteenth centuries to ensure minimal standards of knowledge, these efforts were generally unsuccessful.[12] Instead, medical school diplomas provided accreditation for practitioners. This was insufficient however, with many of the for-profit institutions producing poorly trained physicians who were unqualified to care for patients. The Civil War revealed to the nation's military and political leaders how unfit some of these doctors were and led to a new drive for medical licensing by the states. Starting with Texas in 1873, almost all the states required physicians to have medical licenses in order to practice by 1900. This process boosted physicians in the eyes of the public, with the belief that this certificate vetted the holder as a qualified professional.

State medical licensing necessitated independent examinations to evaluate competency; these were administered by state medical boards, medical societies, or public health agencies. The format could be simple interviews, oral or written exams, and observed patient encounters. In 1916 the National Board of Medical Examiners gave its initial national examination, which was quite extensive and taken on a voluntary basis. It included oral components and essay questions, with practical assessments of laboratory and clinical performance. By 1922 it was shortened and divided into essays on basic science and clinical medicine, along with patient examinations and an oral interrogation. Three decades later, this had evolved into multiple-choice questions, eliminating any subjective bias on the part of the examiners.

Currently, the United States Medical Licensing Examination (USMLE) is required for all individuals who want to practice in the United States. Part 1, which assesses knowledge of the basic medical sciences, is taken after the second year of medical school. Part 2, which focuses on the clinical sciences, is taken during a medical student's senior year. Part 3 occurs after a year or two of clinical training following medical school and analyzes a physician's ability to care for patients and practice medicine without supervision. Since 1999 the USMLE has been computer-based. Foreign medical graduates must also take a special exam (ECFMG) before they can participate in U.S. training programs.

In the early part of the twentieth century, most doctors who functioned as general practitioners took a year of internship after medical school. Surgeons went through additional years of a hospital residency, as did a few medical specialists. As scientific knowledge exploded throughout the twentieth century, longer periods of postgraduate training were felt to be necessary for all medical fields. Residencies were expanded to range from three to five years for most specialties and subspecialties, and occasionally even longer. Fellowships began to be awarded for postresidency training for doctors to develop particular expertise in arcane areas. General practice residencies were also created to allow general practitioners (GPs) to acquire more information and hone their skills. All the specialties and subspecialties now have their own boards that require extensive testing of trainees before they will bestow accreditation. Recertification at defined intervals by these boards is also necessary.

Physicians currently are extensively trained in their fields, with a rigorous medical school curriculum, universal postgraduate training, comprehensive examinations at every level, and stringent standards for licensing. Patients know that all physicians have been well prepared to deliver medical care. Most of the public is not even aware of the term allopathic physicians, as they are the dominant providers of health care and the ones generally identified as physicians.

For most of the twentieth century, physicians were perceived in a positive light by the public; compassionate, caring, and always available for those who were ill or injured, with medical careers a calling for dedicated young men. Continuity, familiarity, and time were the elements that made family physicians so beloved by their patients, with personal contact and face-to-face involvement a big part of the way medicine was practiced. When a patient was sick, doctors would make house calls. Hospitals were utilized only infrequently for surgery or serious illnesses, with most medical care being given at home. Emergency rooms were used mainly for serious trauma cases. The family physician treated every kind of condition—from headaches to heart attacks, pneumonia to ulcers—and also set broken bones and delivered babies. Only the most complicated patients were sent to specialists for consultations, with major surgical problems sent to surgeons. Family practitioners worked largely on their own—rugged individualists using their medical books or journals to solve puzzling cases. Perhaps, occasionally, there would be a phone conversation with another physician to discuss a patient. But medicine was much simpler then, notwithstanding the use of x-rays and advances in surgery, with diagnostic and therapeutic options fairly limited. And in retrospect, the common wisdom used to treat various conditions was often wrong. A prime example was ordering bed rest for three to six weeks after a heart attack. Or three weeks of bed rest for low back problems. Or discouraging physical activity in older people. The knowledge for proper management of many medical conditions was not available.

During much of the twentieth century, medical decisions were also made in a "Father-Knows-Best" manner, which was perhaps one of the consequences of the close relationships physicians had with their patients and families. Doctors were authority figures who told patients what should be done when choices arose, rather than explaining the alternatives and asking for input. In addition, doctors often withheld information they believed might be painful, such as a diagnosis of cancer. Though this impinged on patients' autonomy, it was the way medicine was practiced in the past, and the public was generally accepting of this manner of doing things.

Paradoxically, as medical knowledge has exploded in the last half century, with doctors able to intervene more effectively to help their patients, physicians are no longer held in as high esteem. There are a number of reasons for this. In the new reality of medical practice, there is a shortage of primary care physicians as more doctors have become specialists. And because of time and financial constraints introduced by Medicare and private insurers, physicians have to work faster and see more patients, which means that small talk and "schmoozing" is limited. The knowledge physicians had of their patients and families and the emotional support that was inherent in the doctor-patient relationship has dwindled. In addition, geographic mobility in U.S. society has patients moving frequently and changing doctors, with less continuity of care.

Another factor is that most physicians now practice in groups rather than alone. This has a number of advantages, but does not guarantee that patients will always see the same doctor. It does allow physicians to have coverage and not always be on call. Group practices also provide for the sharing of expenses and administrative staff and economies of scale for many purchases. The groups may be single specialty, multispecialty, or all primary care. They may be large or small, affiliated with hospitals, universities, insurance companies, or unaffiliated. Some group practices have their own hospitals and offer their own health care coverage, and some cover huge geographic areas or have large population bases. A prime example of the latter model is Kaiser Permanente which has a presence in nine states and Washington, D.C.[13] (The largest managed care organization in the United States as of 2006, Kaiser had 8.7 million enrolled members in its health plans, 156,000 employees, 13,727 physicians, 37 medical centers, and 400 medical offices. It generated $34.4 billion in operating revenue, with $1.3 billion net income. While the health plan and hospitals had a not-for-profit status, the medical groups were either professional corporations or for-profit partnerships, depending on their locations.)

The way physicians are compensated now is also different than it was through most of the last century. Previously, doctors were paid a fee directly by the patient, usually at the time of the service. Subsequently, as health insurance became more prevalent, physicians submitted claims to the insurance company (or Medicare) to secure payment, though a proportion of patients still paid directly. As health care costs escalated, more patients were required by their insurance companies to pay a "co-pay" to the physician or provider at the time of service. Currently, over a third of physicians are salaried, working either for hospitals, government, or managed care organizations, and are uninvolved with patient payments. Most of the others are in professional corporations (PCs), where they receive a salary that they themselves determine, plus a proportion of the profits generated after expenses. The PCs receive reimbursement from the insurance companies, the patients, and Medicare, which is used to run the practice and pay the physicians.

The make-up of the physician work force in the United States has also changed dramatically in the last half century, and it impacts the public's perception of doctors as well as the care that is given. International medical graduates comprise an increasing percentage of practicing physicians, with 25 percent of the current first-year residents in U.S. hospitals having graduated from foreign medical schools.[14] Doctors who come from Third World countries may have different notions about physician-patient relationships from what has been fostered here and may be inclined to be more paternalistic when discussing patient concerns. In addition, half the medical students in U.S. schools are women, whose practice objectives may not conform to those of their male colleagues. (Only 72 percent of woman physicians practice full time, compared to 97 percent of men.[15]) And younger physicians in general have different ideas about what they expect from their medical careers than their older peers. Seventy-one percent of physicians under age 50 rated time for their personal lives and family as very important, whereas only 42 percent rated long-term income potential the same way.[16]

Though primary care physicians are better trained and more knowledgeable than in the past, they refer more patients to specialists than ever before. There is just too much information on the diagnosis and treatment of less commonly seen illnesses for any physician who does not specialize in a particular field to master, with the parameters constantly changing. Referral to specialists also occurs with garden-variety conditions that become difficult to treat. The specialists know all the new data on treatment options, new techniques, and new procedures. They also see more patients with the same diagnoses and so are more familiar with their management. But it means that a man with a heart arrhythmia, diabetes, Parkinson's disease, prostate problems and recurrent gastroesophogeal reflux may visit regularly with a cardiologist, endocrinologist, neurologist, urologist and gastroenterologist, in addition to his primary care physician. Though much of this may make sense, it may not make patients happy. In this picture, one can see how the practice of medicine, the doctor-patient relationship, and the cost of medical care has changed. And because fees can be quite high, even though less time is spent with patients, physicians are perceived as mercenary by much of the public, and the respect and affection they previously engendered has diminished.

Medical practices these days also schedule their patients carefully. Many primary care doctors, and almost all specialists, will not see walk-in patients, even in emergencies. Acute problems are told to go to hospital emergency rooms or to walk-in clinics. Many doctors also practice what can be termed "factory-style medicine," with patients given ten-minute time slots and placed in examining rooms by nurses or aides who may take vital signs and document the immediate concerns. Then the physician, who is going from room to room, walks in and quickly assesses the situation with a brief interview and problem-focused examination, orders tests and medication, and sends the patient to an office or desk to have the orders implemented, the bill paid, and a follow-up scheduled if necessary. There is no time for reviewing overall health concerns, for pleasantries, or social conversation. And, of course, house calls are a relic of another era—much too time-consuming and inefficient to be considered. Recently, to expedite communications, many physicians have been using e-mail to receive and send messages. It may work well, but it is a further act of depersonalizing the doctor-patient relationship. (With insurance companies constantly cutting reimbursement for all services, some physicians, who are looking for ways to generate income, are now charging for speaking to patients on the phone, and some are charging for e-mail messages as well.)

As patients' perceptions of physicians, currently, may be less positive than in the past, physicians themselves may be less enthusiastic or even unhappy about the practice of medicine.[17] The reasons for this are numerous. For primary care physicians, the low level of compensation is a major factor. For all physicians, the loss of autonomy can be grating, with insurance companies telling them what they can and can't do. Lifestyle issues weigh on many who may have to spend sixty to eighty hours each week to keep up with their work loads. And much of the work is administrative, trying to get approval for tests, treatments, or medications from insurance companies, addressing denials by insurance companies for various services that have to be appealed, filling out different kinds of reports, and so forth. Physicians say that this not what they signed up for when they went to medical school and trained afterwards, but this is the new reality. Because of the unpleasant work environment, some physicians have left patient care for other types of employment, and others are considering leaving. Of course, this kind of tension and discontent is bound to affect the physician-patient relationship as well.

Whatever the shortcomings about the way medicine is now practiced, it should be remembered that scientific progress has taken medicine to new levels in terms of what can be done for patients, from both a diagnostic and treatment standpoint. Among a number of advances, various kinds of CT scans, MRIs, PET scans, and other types of sophisticated imaging allow physicians to view the interiors of patients' bodies and all the organs noninvasively, locating tumors and other conditions at early stages, which makes treatment potentially more effective. Angiograms are able to assess the status of a person's blood vessels in the heart and throughout the body to determine if surgery, stenting, or other forms of intervention are required. Colonoscopy and endoscopy can document disorders of the gastrointestinal system, while mammography can detect breast cancers. Similarly, new blood tests are able to diagnose cancers, as well as many degenerative and autoimmune diseases, some of which were previously unknown. And potential treatment options have also exploded, including new antibiotics, chemotherapeutic agents, immune-modulating agents, Parkinson's and Alzheimer's drugs, angioplasty and stenting to open up blood vessels, and new operative techniques for a host of conditions. In truth, the list of new treatments is enormous, with many beyond the ken of the generalist, making it imperative for specialists to suggest, prescribe, and monitor many of these options.

(Personalized medicine, using patients' genomic profiles to diagnose diseases, predispositions to diseases, and responses to particular therapies are not yet in widespread use. With new genetic discoveries constantly emerging, the cost of profiling needs to be significantly reduced before this becomes a major element of medical practice, which is bound to happen within a decade or two. As this data could affect people's abilities to obtain health insurance and employment, stringent safeguards of genetic information were implemented in May 2008, when the Genetic Information Nondiscrimination Act was signed into law by President Bush.[18] Some proponents believe that genomic advances provide additional, compelling reasons for universal health coverage, so that an individual's risk is removed from the equation.[19] Stem cell therapy for various conditions is another development that is on the horizon, but as yet does not have significant clinical applications.)

However, the old-fashioned doctor-patient relationship, even with house calls in some instances, is not entirely dead if you can afford to pay for it, as the fees can be extremely steep. Welcome to the world of boutique medicine! In some of the nation's more affluent communities, a new type of medical practice is arising, similar in some aspects to the way family doctors used to function. For this special service, patients pay an annual retainer to the physician (usually an internist) of anywhere from several thousand to ten-thousand dollars or more, to have the doctor available when any medical problems arise. For very wealthy patients, it may be worth it to have your own personal physician on call at all times. (If a boutique doctor has a hundred patients in his or her stable and charges each $5,000 yearly, he or she can make $500,000 a year, unrelated to how often patients are seen. Some boutique doctors also add charges for each visit.) Physicians can greatly limit their practices if they do this, see patients immediately when necessary, spend plenty of time discussing problems with them, and even get to know them and their families. They may also shepherd patients around to specialists and tests to make the process easier and to stay on top of their patients' needs. With so few individuals to care for, doctors find the relationships with them less pressured and more satisfying. These boutique physicians may also have much more free time and a better lifestyle. But from a societal standpoint, this approach only serves to exacerbate the shortage of primary care physicians.

Continuing medical education (CME) requirements are another innovation in the practice of medicine that has developed over the last twenty-five years. Previously, physicians were not mandated to keep their knowledge current, though many did so because they felt it was necessary from an intellectual standpoint or an obligation linked to patient care. But not every physician was disciplined enough to keep abreast of the latest information, even if he or she had good intentions. Now, however, a certain amount of yearly CME is required of doctors by most hospitals to maintain privileges, by some insurance companies to remain participants, and by some states to renew licenses to practice medicine. Most specialty associations also require their members to repeat examinations periodically in order to remain board certified. CME can be obtained by attending meetings and conferences, by reading educational material and taking short exams afterwards, by listening to CDs, or by reading on-line articles or discussions and then being tested.

In addition to this compulsory education, physicians are rarely as isolated as they were in the past. Medical information is always at hand, from the Internet, a plethora of medical journals, hospital meetings, and constant interactions with other doctors. So-called "curbside consults" about patients with other physicians in hospitals or in medical groups are an expected part of current practice.

Patients are also more sophisticated and knowledgeable than they were a half century ago. Aside from generally higher levels of education, patients search the Internet for medical information that is focused on their own conditions. They often come into doctors' offices armed with knowledge (a little of which can be a dangerous thing). The tenor of the times has also changed in terms of how doctors convey information to patients. Partially, because of the threat of malpractice suits, physicians are more forthcoming about every aspect of care, relating the risks and benefits of every choice and every procedure, and often documenting what they have said. Decisions are shared by doctors and their patients after all the pros and cons have been discussed; paternalism is a thing of the past.

Two other unrelated factors that have been changing the practice of medicine are the Health Insurance Portability and Accountability Act (HIPAA) and electronic health records (EHRs). HIPAA was passed by Congress in 1996, with different parts becoming effective from 2003 to 2005.[20] The legislation had a number of objectives. It was supposed to preserve health insurance coverage for employees and their families when jobs were changed or lost and also mandated national standards for electronic health care transactions and claims. In addition, the measure focused on the issue of privacy and security for protected health information (PHI), including medical records and payment information. However, this latter aspect of the law has hindered communication among physicians, between physicians and patients' families, and between health-care facilities and physicians, unless releases have been signed authorizing the transmission of data. (This is obviously not always possible when patients are sick or cognitively impaired.) HIPAA has also added to the administrative overload and costs in all medical offices and medical facilities, with additional forms for patients to sign affirming that they understand HIPAA rules. The legislation has impacted clinical care because of the difficulty in accessing patient data and particularly certain kinds of research. Investigators can't look at patient charts or contact patients for follow-up unless they have previously been granted permission by the patients.

Over the last decade, electronic health records (EHRs—also called electronic medical records, EMRs) have started to be utilized in many physicians' offices with the goal of making care more efficient, less expensive, and safer. Basically, this is the patient's medical chart in an electronic form that is stored on the physician's computer and on a back-up server, or on the Internet. In addition to narrative reports on patient visits, it includes laboratory data, x-ray and other imaging reports, medications used and in use with any adverse reactions, consultations from other physicians, and records of hospitalizations. The EHR is available to the patient's physicians with the use of the proper password. It is easy to visualize the hypothetical value of EHRs, though its potential still remains to be harnessed. So far, only a minority of doctors' offices have installed EHRs and a number of different formats are being employed which can hinder communication among the different systems. And the offices that have EHRs may only be using some of their features. A survey of 2,700 physicians in June 2008 noted that only 4 percent had fully functional EHR systems, while another 13 percent had partial systems, which was behind other industrialized nations.[21] Cost of purchasing and maintaining the equipment was the primary reason more doctors were not using EHRs, along with design problems that hinder usability. (Recently, some insurance companies have been providing bonuses to those medical practices with EHRs.[22]) To be maximally effective, EHRs would have to be standard in all physicians' offices, with all patients' records integrated in the system. This could eliminate duplicate testing and prescribing of medications that had not worked previously or had caused undesirable side effects.

Microsoft introduced a concept in October 2007 called HealthVault, which allows patients to maintain their personal health records on the Web.[23] Initially, the input was to come from the consumers themselves, with the expectation that hospitals, doctors, and other providers could send information to an individual's secure, encrypted file in the future if directed by that person. Doctors or nurses could then access the file with the proper password.

The Internet has also been increasingly employed for prescriptions to be sent directly from doctors' offices to pharmacies, thereby reducing mistakes due to the misinterpretation of physicians' handwriting, patient fraud, and drug abuse (electronic prescribing, or eRx). Eprescribing is mandated by Medicare to be used by all physicians by 2012, or penalties will be imposed.[24] Physicians' charges are also submitted electronically to Medicare and insurance companies, which greatly simplifies the process.

When health care reform is enacted, it must include the universal use by physicians of electronic health records to improve the quality of care and lower costs.

Practicing medicine in the twenty-first century will be a quantum leap from the twentieth century, with even newer diagnostic tests available, new treatment options, new ways to keep records, and enhanced communication between physicians.

## Organized Medicine and Health Care Reform Efforts

As mentioned, establishing authority and legitimacy in the eyes of the public were major concerns for physicians early on in the United States. Insecurity in social status and earning power was particularly prevalent in the middle ranks of the medical profession, mostly younger men who did not come from the best families or graduate from the best schools, and who felt economically vulnerable.[25] Organizing the profession was seen by many of these physicians as a path to legitimacy and a way to achieve preeminence over rival health care "experts," with the licensing of practitioners as one of their important objectives.

County and state medical societies were formed in the early 1800s in a number of regions. In many instances, state legislatures allowed these societies, along with some of the medical schools, to grant licenses to physicians to practice.[26] However, there were no uniform criteria, and personal contacts and influence played an important role in licensure. By the 1840s, there was a desire among some ambitious young physicians in New York and other cities to create a national medical organization that could work towards developing standards for accreditation and could wield political power in the battle against alternative health care competitors. In 1847, delegates from state medical societies and medical colleges convened in Philadelphia and formed the American Medical Association (AMA), which had its first official meeting the following year in Baltimore.[27]

For the remainder of the nineteenth century, however, the AMA was unsuccessful in attaining its intended objectives and was far from the powerhouse its founders had envisioned. Alternative medical practitioners flourished throughout the nation as new and unproven methods of care found adherents among the populace. Though this was during a time of great progress in medical science, which enhanced allopathic physicians' ability to treat various conditions, public credibility lagged behind. Attempts to reform medical education during this period failed, as medical schools insisted on remaining sovereign entities, refusing to conform to externally set standards by bodies like the AMA. In addition to those medical schools that generally adhered to orthodox teaching, there were a number that espoused unscientific practices and graduated homeopathic doctors, eclectics, and Thomasonians to minister to the public.[28] The press, the courts, and the legislatures that weighed competing claims from the different schools of medical thought were unsure of their validity and were content to let the doctors battle among themselves.

The AMA was also weak, lacked an authoritative voice, and had minimal financial resources, no permanent structure, and a limited membership within the profession. (The AMA had only 8,000 members as of 1900, with the combined membership of the national, state, and local medical societies reaching 33,000, which was less than one-third of the total 110,000 practicing physicians.[29]) AMA delegates, representing medical societies, hospitals, and medical schools, met once a year to debate issues of common concern, with members then retreating to their home bases and generating little follow-through on the association's proposals. Political battles also caused fractures within the group, with some members splitting off to form rival organizations. In speaking about this era, Paul Starr noted in *The Social Transformation of American Medicine*: "Professional organizations languished because they had no leverage over individual doctors. The medical practitioners in the nineteenth century could get by pretty much on their own. They did not need access to hospital facilities, since very little medical care took place there. The natural inclination of physicians then was to solve their problems individually."[30]

Shortly after the turn of the twentieth century, realizing that the fight against alternative practitioners had been both damaging and futile, the AMA revised its code of ethics and no longer prohibited relations between regular physicians and their competitors. This allowed homeopathic and eclectic physicians to join state and local medical societies, thereby blurring the lines between the different kinds of doctors. Though this change may have instilled some degree of legitimacy on alternative practitioners, it heralded the end of their public popularity, as they were no longer seen as heretics persecuted by organized medicine and deserving of sympathy. The general population had also become more aware of the great advances in medical science and was more willing to entrust itself to trained (and licensed) physicians. Homeopathic and eclectic medical schools quickly dwindled and disappeared. However, new medical sects that challenged orthodox scientific tenets arose to replace them, including osteopaths, chiropractors, and Christian scientists, the latter rejecting all medical intervention in favor of prayer as a treatment for illnesses.

Structural reorganization by the AMA in 1901 further strengthened it, as well as its state and local medical associations. The AMA was transformed into a confederation of state medical societies, the latter of which were to be assembled from a confederation of local societies. From that point on, to join a medical society at any level, physicians had to pay dues and join all levels. With greater financial resources and increased membership, state societies were now more able to influence state legislatures about issues that affected medical practice, particularly laws involving the licensing of physicians. State and local medical societies also attracted members because they were a bulwark against malpractice suits. This was particularly important because "standard of care" in a locality was the criterion used by the courts to judge whether or not physicians had committed malpractice, and society members could testify as to what that standard was.

On a national level, the AMA became a skillful instrument representing physicians' interests in Washington. Growing from 8,000 members in 1900 to 70,000 in 1910, the organization was able to claim it represented half the nation's physicians, eventually reaching 60 percent in 1920.[31] The AMA backed the recommendations of the Flexner report in 1910 which described the needed reforms in the nation's medical schools and helped to get them implemented.[32] In the 1920s, the AMA also developed standards for the training of medical specialists and determined which hospitals had the resources to train them. By this time, the AMA had become extremely powerful politically as well, and was opposed to "any plan embodying the system of compulsory insurance . . . controlled or regulated by any state or the federal government."[33] Organized medicine was now a force that had to be considered by Congress and any executive agencies with oversight functions connected to health care. It was also a force resistant to change. Throughout the remainder of the twentieth century, the AMA played a dominant role in rejecting and resisting any health care reform measures that envisioned government participation.

The idea of national health insurance was raised initially by Theodore Roosevelt in 1912 as part of his Progressive Party platform, and it followed the lead of several European nations, including Germany. Nothing came of it until the 1930s when it was reintroduced in the context of the Depression. However, consistently suspicious of government control, the AMA battled against these programs. Indeed, the 1935 Social Security Act was passed without comprehensive health insurance because of resistance and perseverance by the AMA, even though the time had seemed right for this measure.[34] (The AMA's opposition kept health care reform off the table for another ten years.) Also during the 1930s, the AMA tried to block its members from participating in rudimentary HMOs that were created in an attempt to deliver affordable health care.[35] Because of this, the AMA was cited in 1943 by the Supreme Court for violation of the Sherman Antitrust Act. Physician membership grew steadily during this period, topping 100,000 in 1936.

The next attempt at systemic health care reform occurred after World War II when Harry Truman proposed compulsory health insurance that would be funded by a payroll deduction. Again, the time seemed fortuitous, but the AMA mounted a vigorous lobbying effort and was successful in defeating the bill. In an era when Communism was a fearsome enemy, the AMA labeled the concept of government involvement in health care as "socialized medicine," and made it seem as if it were a Communist plot to undermine the free market system. When Truman won an upset victory in 1948 to remain president, the AMA established "a special assessment of members to resist enslavement of the medical profession."[36] During the remainder of the 1940s and the 1950s, the AMA was able to defeat every attempt to enact Medicare legislation and national health insurance, thus acquiring "an aura of invincibility"[37] in Washington. Its opposition to these proposals utilized public-relations and lobbying firms in far-reaching campaigns, more extensively than anything seen previously. The American Medical Political Action Committee (AMPAC) was formed in the early 1960s to support friendly candidates, with the AMA giving financial backing solely to those hostile to Medicare.

John Kennedy ran for president in 1960 with a platform calling for health care benefits for older Americans under Social Security. After his election, health insurance became his top domestic issue as part of the New Frontier, with the AMA standing strongly against its passage. Though Kennedy was not able to see it enacted before his assassination, Johnson took the ball and ran with it after his landslide victory in 1964, which also gave him a large Democratic majority in Congress. Johnson, a superb political tactician, was able to shepherd the bill through Congress with Southern conservatives and Republicans as adversaries. In 1965, Medicare was finally passed by Congress and signed into law by Johnson, providing hospitalization benefits and payments for physician services for the aged, with the package being even more generous than its advocates had hoped for.[38] Medicaid, providing health benefits for the poor, was also enacted.

To lessen AMA opposition and to encourage physician participation in Medicare, doctors were allowed to continue to charge their usual, customary, and reasonable fees, with Medicare paying a fixed amount for the services, and physicians being permitted to bill patients for the rest. However, under this system, payments from Medicare to physicians escalated annually during the 1970s and 1980s at an average rate of more than 14 percent,[39] which was clearly unsustainable. In addition, there were imbalances in the amounts going to specialists and primary care doctors, being particularly disproportionate for surgical and diagnostic services. There were regional variances as well, which were locked in place by the method being employed for reimbursement.

To try and achieve more equity, and hopefully reduce the growth in Medicare spending, Congress mandated the Physician Payment Review Commission in the mid-1980s to restructure the payment system. The panel's recommendations were enacted in the Omnibus Budget Reconciliation Act of 1989, which was to go into effect in 1992. Medicare payments were henceforth to be determined by a Resource Based Relative Value Scale (RBRVS), with physicians billing their services based on the current procedural terminology (CPT) codes. The RBRVS for each CPT code was to be determined by three factors: (1) physician work (time, skill, and training), (2) practice expense, and (3) malpractice expense. It was then to be adjusted by region to determine reimbursement. The 1989 legislation also set limits on the amounts that doctors could bill Medicare patients beyond the authorized fees; this became known as balanced billing, and tied growth in physicians' fees to spending targets that were determined in advance. Yet since then, time and again, pressure by organized medicine has been able to get Congress to rescind any scheduled cuts in physician reimbursement when Medicare spending targets were exceeded.[40] And there has been no movement by Congress to correct the flaws in the original formula and produce a long term solution for physician payments.[41]

Since the law's enactment, there has been a significant slowing in the yearly increase in physician reimbursement, and many of the commercial insurance companies are also using this formula to calculate their payments to physicians. But physicians (as well as hospitals and other providers) have learned how to game the system by changing coding and diagnoses to improve reimbursement, with specialty associations and private ventures giving seminars and sending out bulletins to train physicians on how to maximize their payments.[42] As reimbursement for services has remained fairly static, physicians have also considerably increased the volume of their services in order to maintain their income.[43] (It is also true that Medicare's reimbursement has not kept pace with increased overhead expenses in physicians' offices.) However, there continues to be disproportionate payment for imaging and procedures under the RBRVS, with medical and surgical specialists and radiologists being favored over primary care physicians.

After the passage of Medicare, opposition for the most part became muted, with the program attaining immense popularity and its benefits becoming politically sacrosanct. Politicians realized they would pay a price at election time if they did not embrace Medicare. Not only did it permit the elderly to obtain health care without facing impoverishment or asking their children for help, but it brought a measure of respect to older people who were now able to pay for the services they used.

Family bonds between generations were strengthened as the elderly were less dependent on their children. The health status of seniors also improved significantly as they were no longer afraid to seek medical help for acute illnesses or chronic conditions. All Americans now expect Medicare to be there for them when they reach the age threshold, or if they become disabled, and use this knowledge in their financial planning. (In 2003, it was estimated that 35 million older Americans and 6 million disabled were covered by Medicare.[44])

Besides the programs' effect on individual lives, Medicare and Medicaid have also had a profound impact on the entire health care system in the United States. The new income generated by these programs allowed hospitals across the nation to modernize their facilities and purchase up-to-date equipment, thus enhancing patient care. In addition, it supported the development of academic medical centers with even more advanced technology, which were able to provide specialized care to select patients and perform medical research. Funds from these programs have also been a mainstay of residency programs in hospitals and academic centers, thereby helping to train various kinds of physicians.

Interestingly, although organized medicine fought tooth and nail against Medicare, its leaders subsequently realized that physicians were benefiting greatly from the program, their lack of foresight not withstanding. Doctors were suddenly being paid by patients who were previously being seen for free, or at reduced fees, or who went to clinics for their health care. Physicians' incomes, as well as their patient loads, increased significantly. Since the advent of Medicare, the AMA has not tried to eliminate it, but has instead battled continuously for increases in physician fees. Yet the AMA still fights against any possible expansion of the program, such as one to cover all American citizens in a single-payer system. An article in the *Journal of the American Medical Association* in January 2008 points out that social justice in providing health care to all, and improving the quality of medical care, has never been a priority for organized medicine, whose main concern has been its members' financial interests.[45]

Since the passage of Medicare, attempts to develop a comprehensive national health insurance plan continued in the early 1970s, with the unions in the forefront and Senator Edward Kennedy as its leading proponent.[46] In spite of opposition from the AMA, with broad Congressional and public backing, President Richard Nixon signed on and his administration formulated a bill that was sent to Congress. But attempts to craft legislation acceptable to liberals and moderates in both political parties stalled and then died after Watergate and the Nixon resignation. Under Jimmy Carter, another plan for expansion of health care coverage went nowhere when it was attacked by organized medicine, business, and conservatives. During the Reagan-Bush administrations from 1981 to 1993, health care reform fell by the wayside, even as the number of uninsured continued to increase.

(The AMA's unrelenting opposition from the outset to government-sponsored national health insurance can at least partially be explained by the disproportionate representation of surgeons and surgical subspecialists in the organization's hierarchy. This group of physicians have always been higher earners than their medical brethren and had more to lose financially if national health insurance came to fruition, restricting fees or imposing physician salaries. As surgeons also tend to work fewer hours than primary care physicians, they had more time available to become involved in medical politics. In addition, they were able to schedule elective procedures at their convenience, which allowed them to attend meetings and participate in AMA activities without a significant loss of income. They had both the motivation and the time. More recently, surgical fees have been curtailed under RBRVS and high malpractice premiums have cut into surgeon's incomes.)

Bill Clinton chose health care reform as his signal issue in the 1992 presidential campaign, and when elected, appointed his wife Hillary to devise a program and get it enacted. But their Health Security plan, using "managed competition," was so complicated and had so many layers of administration that it was easy for the coalition of interests against it, including the AMA and the health insurance industry, to defeat the bill. Though the "Harry and Louise" advertisements by the opponents of the Clintons' health care plan were felt to have played a decisive role in its demise, the lack of a well-organized constituency pushing for its passage, as the elderly had done with Medicare, and poor political management of the bill were probably just as responsible.

After the debacle of the Clinton efforts for health care reform, the next Congressional foray into health care was through the Balanced Budget Act of 1997. Included in this bill was the concept of Medicare + Choice, which subsequently became known as the Medicare Advantage Plan (Medicare Part C). This was envisioned by conservatives as a way to get seniors to enroll in private insurance plans, by giving them extra benefits, including prescription drug coverage, lower or no copayments, and the elimination of supplementary coverage. Its backers believed that Medicare would be transformed by this new legislation bringing "competition, choice and market dynamics into the program."[47] Patients in these managed care plans had to go to certain doctors and designated hospitals for their care, and the insurance companies offering these plans were paid a fixed rate by Medicare for each enrollee, no matter what services were utilized.

However, the insurance companies that developed these plans found them to be more expensive than regular Medicare (about 12 percent on average[48]) and began to abandon them, raise premiums, or cut benefits. Indeed, many plans were discontinued by the companies because they were unprofitable, confusing those people who had enrolled. To stem the tide on what could be considered a failed program, the Bush administration stepped into the breach, agreeing to give subsidies to these private insurance plans to keep them in business and pushing the Medicare Modernization Act through Congress. (Medicare now pays Medicare Advantage plans an average of 13 percent more for services than regular Medicare, and some even more.[49]) Though more than 9 million Medicare beneficiaries are currently members of Medicare Advantage plans (roughly one in five Medicare enrollees[50]), it seems to make little economic sense for the government to be paying more for enrollees in these plans that were originally conceived as a way to control costs through the market. (Advocates of these plans point to the fact that enrollees are getting more benefits than under traditional Medicare. However, critics assert that the insurance companies tend to "cherry pick" the younger and healthier seniors for their plans, leaving the older, less healthy seniors, such as nursing home patients, as the responsibility of traditional Medicare.)

Medicare Part D, partial prescription drug coverage, was the next major piece of health care legislation, which was passed by a Republican Congress in 2003 as part of the Medicare Modernization Act, becoming effective in 2006. With organized medicine essentially on the sidelines for this bill, and a number of conservatives behind it, the legislation was able to make its way through Congress in spite of its enormous cost. Though it does help many seniors pay for their drugs, many others are unhappy with some of the bill's features. This includes the donut hole for reimbursement, where enrollees have to pay completely for their medications (after spending $2,510 in 2008 up to $4050), high copayments for some prescriptions, increasing premiums, and the need to switch some medications. Expenditures for Medicare Part D in 2007 amount to 11.6 percent of the total Medicare budget ($50 billion out of $432 billion).[51] However, it is estimated that Medicare Part D alone will be responsible for 1 percent of the nation's GDP in less than twenty years as drug expenses balloon.[52] Unless better cost constraints are built into Medicare spending, including part D, the unfunded liabilities of the program will soar.

Notwithstanding its opposition to comprehensive health care reform throughout the twentieth century, the AMA did a number of positive things from a public health standpoint. These include its recommendation for polio vaccinations in 1960, its emphasis on the dangers of cigarette smoking, pushing for the mandatory use of seat belts for children, fighting discrimination against AIDS patients, pushing to raise the drinking age to twenty-one, favoring a patient's bill of rights, and so forth. It has also published a weekly medical journal, the *Journal of the American Medical Association* (JAMA), along with many influential specialty journals, which have produced important articles on medical research and health care issues. In addition, the AMA has championed malpractice reform through the years, but its efforts in this area so far have been unsuccessful. It has been fighting against an even more powerful lobbying group in this crusade, the American Trial Lawyers Association, which has many natural allies in Congress, where many of its members themselves are lawyers.

Though AMA membership increased throughout most of the twentieth century, a report in 2005 showed that it had dropped during the previous fifteen years.[53] The report noted that less than one in three U.S. physicians were members, 244,500 of 850,000. (The British Medical Association has about 80 percent of physicians as members.) Various reasons have been cited for the decline, including its inability to find ways to get coverage for the uninsured, the lack of movement on malpractice reform, and its failure to address other issues of importance to physicians. Nevertheless, the AMA still remains the dominant voice of U.S. medicine and its major organized force.

## CHAPTER 3

# EVOLUTION OF THE AMERICAN HEALTH CARE SYSTEM

## Hospitals, the Health Insurance Industry, the Pharmaceutical Industry, and the Medical Device Industry

Nothing is more free than the imagination of man; and though it cannot exceed that original stock of ideas furnished by the internal and external senses, it has unlimited power of mixing, compounding, separating, and dividing these ideas, in all the varieties of fiction and vision.

—David Hume, *Enquiries Concerning Human Understanding*[1]

## The Evolution of Hospitals

At the beginning of the nineteenth century, the practice of medicine provided little in the way of treatment options for serious illnesses. The hospital and almshouse (or pesthouse) were the places designated by society for its diseased members, specifically its impoverished lower classes, to reside during an illness and usually to die. These institutions were unsanitary, overcrowded, repellent habitats used only by those individuals whose families could not care for them. For most people of even meager means, dying at home was the norm, with the physician (or clergyman) being the agent of solace for the patient and family, but unable to intervene in the process.

Paul Starr noted in *The Social Transformation of American Medicine* (1982) that, "before the last hundred years, hospitals and medical practice had relatively little to do with each other. From their earliest origins in preindustrial societies, hospitals had been primarily religious and charitable institutions for tending the sick, rather than medical institutions for their cure. . . . The reconstitution of the hospital involved its redefinition as an institution of medical science rather than of social welfare, its reorganization on the lines of a business rather than a charity, and its reorientation to professionals and their patients rather than to patrons and the poor."[2]

From its role as a repository for the poor and sick, over the last century and a half, hospitals have evolved into modern temples of health care with vast arrays of diagnostic and therapeutic modalities to evaluate and treat patients. The metamorphosis began with an initial surge of growth from 1870 to 1910, with the number of hospitals in the United States soaring from 178 in the year 1873, to more than 4,300 in 1909.[3] Several developments propelled this increase: the use of anesthesia for surgery, the control of infection with aseptic techniques and the use of antiseptics, and the training of professional nurses to provide care. There were now reasons for sick people to go to the hospital. Something could be done to help them.

The period after World War II until about 1980 was another time of hospital expansion. Small rural hospitals were built with financing under the Hill-Burton Act, and many of the older hospitals modernized their plants, acquired new technology, and added new beds. Funds came from Medicare, Medicaid, and the increased number of people with health insurance. Since 1980, however, hospital occupancy rates have gone down significantly due to pressures for cost containment, the prospective payment system for Medicare patients, and greater delivery of services on an outpatient basis. From 1990 to 1995, the number of hospital beds in the United States declined from 927,000 to 830,000.[4] Hospital occupancy rates were 76 percent in 1980, decreasing to 63 percent in 1990, even with fewer beds. Notwithstanding this contraction, the costs for each day of hospital care and for all hospital services continued to escalate each year. Of the total U.S. health care expenditures of $2.1 trillion in 2006, about 31 percent, $648 billion, went for hospital care and services.

The prospective payment system that was instituted by Medicare in the 1980s reimbursed the hospital a fixed amount for each patient admitted, based on his or her diagnosis-related group (DRG), rather than per hospital day and services performed. The sum paid was the same no matter how complicated the care, or how long the hospital stay might be. Hospitals that were most efficient in discharging patients early, or had patients that were less sick, could profit more from these patients. And to maximize their reimbursement, hospitals optimized the DRG codes they submitted (using codes that generated more income), with those that did a better job able to obtain more money.[5] From 1985 to 1999, with fewer patients admitted, the average length of stay went from 7.1 to 5 days, a major decline in the utilization of hospital beds.[6] With the drop in occupancy rates, hospitals sought new sources of income and found them in ambulatory care. Revenues from outpatient visits and procedures, which were virtually nil prior to 1985, were responsible for

30–50 percent of revenues in community hospitals in 1999, with the number of outpatient visits jumping by 89 percent.[7] In 1980, only 16 percent of surgical procedures in community hospitals were performed on outpatients. This grew to 62 percent in 1999. In addition to ambulatory surgical centers, hospitals developed walk-in medical centers apart from their campuses, outpatient diagnostic centers, and rehabilitation facilities. Some of these were created as joint ventures with physician participation.

Traditionally, there have been three power centers competing for control within U.S. community hospitals: the Board of Trustees, the medical staff, and the administration. In the nineteenth century, the Boards were dominant, with individuals who donated funds to sustain the institutions determining how they were to be run, the staffing, and even the patients who were admitted. To a large degree, the medical staff supplanted the Board in the first half of the twentieth century, governing the admission of patients and what services were to be used, thus controlling hospital finances. Over the last 40 or so years, the medical staff's power has gradually eroded, with the hospital administration now in the ascendancy. The hiring of full-time, salaried physicians by most hospitals has further bolstered the control of the administration, weakening the medical staff's position. In addition to resident physicians who are being trained, hospitals now have full-time, salaried physicians working in the emergency rooms, intensivists in the ICUs, hospitalists managing patients on the wards, radiologists, pathologists, and anesthesiologists. (Some of these physicians may only be partially salaried and have other sources of income, such as fee-for-service.) Many hospitals also employ salaried specialists, such as department heads of medicine, surgery, pediatrics, obstetrics, and so forth. In addition, they may hire surgeons, cardiologists, neurologists, and gastroenterologists for hospital work. Some institutions have their own managed care plans and pay both primary care physicians and subspecialists to provide services for their enrollees. In 2006, 18 percent of working physicians in the United States, or 114,000 physicians, were employed by hospitals.[8]

Hospitals in the United States today occupy the entire spectrum in terms of size, sophistication, and staffing. Orientation and mission also vary, depending on their origins, location, funding, and various other factors. Their commonality lies in caring for people who are ill. Among the different types of institutions are university hospitals, large community hospitals, small community hospitals, for-profit hospitals, specialty hospitals, and psychiatric hospitals.

University hospitals are believed to provide the most sophisticated medical care available. They usually possess the most advanced technology and have experts on their staffs from every field because of their medical school connections. These hospitals are used to train medical students, interns, and residents and to conduct clinical research. Though attending physicians nominally care for the patients, a major role is played by the house staff. In addition to routine patients, the most challenging diagnostic and treatment problems are sent to these hospitals with the hope that the body of university specialists and subspecialists can find answers and provide effective management. Research may be as important to these physicians as clinical care, which may allow patients opportunities to obtain experimental treatments for rare illnesses or for conditions that have not responded to conventional therapy. Excessive consultations and evaluations may be part of this picture along with multiple examinations by students and house staff. Although the technology and treatment at university hospitals is usually at the cutting edge of medical science, care may be costly and impersonal.

Large community hospitals are for the most part voluntary institutions supported by the communities, religious bodies, or charitable groups. Many of these hospitals were originally established by physicians and community members who perceived a need for them. The larger centers often deliver a high level of patient care, rated a notch below the university institutions. Some of these community hospitals have training programs for house staff, as well as the latest technology, and are able to attract competent, young physicians to their catchment areas to practice. The top hospitals in this group may also have medical school affiliations, which helps with education and patient care. Though attending physicians in the community previously directed the care of their patients in the hospital, this task now falls increasingly on the shoulders of the hospitalists and intensivists. The presence of house officers, who are always available in the hospital and engaged with attendings about patient management, is considered to contribute to better patient care.

Smaller community hospitals serve a smaller population base in rural areas and have less advanced technology and no house staff. They may be voluntary, under the aegis of state or local governments, or are for-profit, and are generally less than a hundred beds. Because doctors may not always be present within the confines of these hospitals, physician's assistants (PAs) may be used on the wards or in the ERs for routine care and triage. Many of these hospitals have closed in the last few decades and many others are not financially viable. Often these institutions are used to stabilize seriously ill patients initially, then transfer them to larger hospitals for more definitive care.

Municipal and county hospitals are government supported, with additional funding from patients covered by Medicaid, Medicare, or private insurance. Some of these institutions have trauma centers with special teams to deal with major injuries, particularly from motor vehicle accidents and gunshot wounds, though many of their patients lack insurance and are unable to pay for this expensive care. The patient mix in municipal hospitals includes the indigent, the elderly, and the uninsured, with a smattering of others. Because of funding problems, the physical plants are sometimes inadequate and the technology limited, with understaffing by nurses, aides, and technicians. However, these hospitals are an important cog in the health care machine, dealing disproportionately with the problems of poverty, including drug and alcohol abuse, AIDS, trauma, and the complications of diabetes and hypertension. With political appointees on the administrative staffs and boards of these institutions, politics may affect their performance. Medical school affiliation has been obtained by some of these hospitals to help in recruiting house staff and attendings and to improve quality. A number of these hospitals in major cities have been forced to close because they were losing money and providing suboptimal care, the two factors interrelated. An infusion of funding from health care reform could make a positive difference for many of these institutions.

Large state psychiatric hospitals that once incarcerated significant numbers of psychotic patients are mostly out of business since the advent of psychotropic medications. Many of these patients are now followed in outpatient clinics or seen by caseworkers in their homes, to be certain they are taking their prescribed drugs. If acute hospitalization is needed, the patients are admitted to the psychiatric wards of community or municipal hospitals, generally for short stays to adjust their medications. Small, freestanding psychiatric hospitals generally serve a more affluent clientele, or at least patients with adequate insurance, and usually deal with drug and alcohol addiction as well. These may be either voluntary or for-profit in nature. There are also institutions that manage drug and alcohol problems only.

Veterans Administration hospitals (VA) have recently received bad press because of the problems wounded soldiers encountered when they returned to the United States. However, most of the difficulties were in the military hospitals such as Walter Reed, rather than the VAs. In general, the quality of care and patient satisfaction at the VA hospitals has been quite good, both for in-patient and out-patient services, and delivered at a lower cost than at other health centers (as noted in Chapter 1). If problems exist with the new arrivals, it may be related to a lack of adequate funding from the federal government to handle the surge of severely injured men and women from Iraq and Afghanistan who require a host of medical, surgical, psychiatric, and rehabilitative services.

For-profit, investor-owned hospitals, comprised 13 percent of the 5,810 hospitals in the United States in 2002, according to the American Hospital Association.[9] Private hospitals first came into existence in small numbers during the middle of the last century. They were mostly physician owned and had limited impact on overall health care (often, they were started by surgeons who wanted a place to operate that they could control). Currently, however, for-profit hospitals are usually links in chains of institutions owned and operated by large corporations, which deliver care to a significant segment of the U.S. population. These hospitals are most prevalent in the sunbelt regions (including the southeast, southwest, and California) and less so in the northeast. Two of the largest for-profit hospital chains are Hospital Corporation of America (HCA) and Tenet Health Care. According to its Web site in June 2008, HCA owned and operated 169 hospitals and 109 freestanding surgical centers in 20 states and London, England. Financial statistics on the company were not available, as the corporation had been taken private in a leveraged buyout in 2006. Tenet Health Care's Web site stated that it had 53 acute care hospitals in twelve states, with over 14,000 licensed beds and 62,000 employees. In addition, it had ancillary health care businesses, including ambulatory surgical centers and diagnostic imaging facilities. Their net operating revenue was $8.7 billion in fiscal year 2007.

For-profit hospitals are what their name describes: institutions whose objective is to make a profit for stockholders or private investors (which also translates into increased compensation for their executives). Due to high executive pay and tax obligations, because they are profit-making, the operating costs of these hospitals are greater than at nonprofit institutions. The major concern at these businesses is the bottom line, rather than the quality of patient care (as will be shown). Their executives are willing to cut corners to cut costs when delivering care, as a number of reports have confirmed. For-profit hospitals spend less on personnel, avoid charity patients, and shorten patients' stays to lower their costs.[10] Studies in the past have also shown 6–7 percent higher death rates at for-profit hospitals than at nonprofit institutions.[11] Another study noted an increased risk of death of 2 percent in for-profit hospitals, indicating that 14,000 people who die annually at these hospitals would have lived if they had been treated at nonprofits.[12] Rates of postoperative complications and preventable adverse events were also higher at for-profit hospitals than nonprofits.[13]

In addition to poorer outcomes for patients, the care provided at for-profit hospitals is costlier than at other institutions. One study showed that Medicare spending per capita in areas served by for-profit hospitals was 10–15 percent higher than in areas served by nonprofits, as was the rate of increase in spending.[14] One apparent reason for this was that investor-owned hospitals charged 19 percent more for their services than nonprofits.[15] Of $37 billion spent at these for-profit hospitals for care in 2001, $6 billion could have been saved if they had been nonprofit institutions.[16] For-profit hospitals were found to upcode the DRGs of their patients for Medicare billing in a higher percentage of admissions than nonprofits, in order to increase their reimbursement.[17] In fact, both HCA and Tenet Health Care were convicted of fraudulent billing practices (among other charges) in the past and had to pay hefty fines (discussed in section on fraud in Chapter 4).

(For-profit ownership of dialysis units was also associated with increased mortality compared to nonprofits, believed to result from economic pressures to cut costs and delays in placing patients for renal transplants in order to maintain them as a source of income.[18])

For-profit hospitals are another example of why market-based solutions will not work in health care reform. In the pursuit of profits, some executives will try to game the system in legal ways, but will resort to unethical and illegal practices to increase their company's earnings (and their own compensation). And not only does it cost more, but patient care suffers.

Specialty hospitals devoted to cardiac, orthopedic, women's conditions, or surgical procedures are a small segment of the hospital mix, but have been increasing in number. In 2003, there were one hundred of these specialty hospitals in the United States, with 26 more in the planning or construction stages.[19] Seventy-four percent were for-profit and about one-third were owned by chains. Two-thirds of the specialty hospitals were in just seven states: California, Texas,

Arizona, Louisiana, Oklahoma, Kansas, and South Dakota. There are several concerns about these institutions. One is that they skim off the more profitable patients and leave the rest to the general hospitals. They also tend to focus on the most profitable procedures and admit patients that are less severely ill or have less complicated conditions, leaving the sicker, higher-cost patients dependent on the general hospitals. Given the fixed payments that Medicare and the insurance companies use to reimburse hospitals by discharge diagnoses (DRG system), the favorable patient selection by the specialty hospitals helps them financially, while placing a greater burden on the general hospitals. Another concern is that the specialty hospitals provide less emergency care, which usually includes more poor people and the uninsured.

Questions have also been raised about physician ownership of these hospitals and what appear to be conflicts of interest. Seventy percent of specialty hospitals have some degree of ownership by physicians, either individually or as a part of a group, with the ownership percentage averaging slightly over 50 percent.[20] Financial incentives for these owner-physicians presents the potential of altered referral patterns and/or orders for additional tests or services. (Legislation which is currently on the books, that is supposed to reduce physician self-referral, does not seem to cover this area.) Despite complaints from the general hospitals that the specialty hospitals are hurting them, there have been few restrictions upon them and they seem to be thriving. Though a number of bills were proposed and passed in either one or the other houses of Congress in the last session to prohibit physicians from referring Medicare or Medicaid patients to hospitals in which they have a financial interest, none of them passed both houses to become law.[21] The measure was supported by the American Hospital Association, but opposed by the AMA and the Bush White House. (One of the problems was that several senators placed earmarks into the bills protecting specific hospitals in their states from its provisions, instead of allowing the law to be applied universally.)

## The Health Insurance Industry

Though Theodore Roosevelt and his Progressives suggested the creation of national health insurance in 1912, it was not a burning issue for most Americans. At the beginning of the twentieth century, health care costs were low and hospital expenses were generally not a concern. There was actually greater worry about the possibility of lost wages due to illness, and families bought "sickness insurance" to replace the income that would be missed if the breadwinner became sick. Most commercial insurance companies did not even offer health insurance policies, as they did not believe there was a large enough market for them. Those private insurance plans that did exist were fairly limited in scope, providing direct service to employees in specific industries, with the patient being unable to choose either physician or hospital, and no indemnity of costs if a patient went outside the system.

By the 1920s, knowledge of the scientific advances in medicine had become widespread, and licensure seemed to indicate better quality of care by physicians. More people began to seek medical help when they were ill, with increasing urbanization also making physicians more available to the population. However, as health care costs began to rise and Americans began to be hospitalized more frequently, it became difficult for working families to manage the expenses associated with illnesses and trauma. Organized labor championed proposals for compulsory health insurance in several states during this period, but no legislation was ever passed.[22] President Franklin Roosevelt's failure to include national health insurance as part of his Social Security program in the 1930s opened the way for other methods of health care coverage to be formulated.

The first insurance plans that gained public acceptance appeared during the early 1930s and paid for hospital care. These were sponsored by groups of hospitals and were nonprofit. During the Depression, hospital use had fallen off as most people were unable to afford the costs. Hospitals saw insurance as a way to regain patients. Their executives administered and controlled these plans, which had their own territories and state regulations, and were noncompetitive. The plans later combined and evolved into Blue Cross under the aegis of the American Hospital Association (AHA). Blue Cross guidelines reduced price competition among hospitals and allowed enrollees free choice of hospitals and physicians.[23] The enabling legislation in various states for Blue Cross maintained their tax-exempt status as nonprofit organizations and freed them from insurance regulations, such as reserve requirements.

Insurance coverage for physicians developed separately from the hospital plans and was slower to reach fruition. Physicians wanted their plans to be given the same tax advantages as Blue Cross, but remain under physician control. The first prepayment plan that covered physicians' services began in California in 1939, with other state medical societies sponsoring their own plans. In 1946, the different plans affiliated and were subsequently marketed as Blue Shield. Most of these plans paid a fixed amount for physician services, with patients responsible for the remainder of the charges. This allowed physicians the freedom to set their own fees. (At that time, many physicians charged patients differently based on their assessment of the patient's ability to pay.) However, some of these plans reimbursed physicians for their services using an established payment schedule, without additional charges permitted.

When commercial insurers became aware of the success of Blue Cross and Blue Shield, they began to seek the same business with their own products. But employers were generally uninterested in providing health insurance to their workers during the 1930s, a time when unemployment was rife and it was easy finding new employees. This attitude began to change during World War II when the federal government instituted wage controls during a period of inflation, and it was difficult for companies to attract workers.[24] Since the government placed no restrictions on the benefits that might be offered, businesses used health insurance to recruit and retain workers. The employer-based plans became even more enticing with government rulings that health insurance was not subject to taxes, and that benefits such as health insurance could be negotiated by unions as part of their wage packages. (Government tax benefits subsidizing employer-based health insurance were valued at $188 billion in 2004, equivalent to almost $1,200 for each participant in these plans.[25])

Commercial insurance companies were successful in the health care market despite Blue Cross and Blue Shield's head start, because the Blues had nonprofit status and were forced to use community rating for their policies. This meant that all subscribers had to be charged the same amount when they purchased coverage, whether they were healthy or had preexisting conditions. The commercial insurance companies were able to use experience rating for those who enrolled, offering lower premiums to healthy individuals or relatively healthy groups, whereas those with health issues were charged more or even rejected.[26] By cherry-picking their subscribers, the commercial companies were able to generate substantial profits and rapidly expand their subscriber base.

In the decade from 1940 to 1950, the number of enrollees in all private health insurance plans climbed from 20.6 million to 143.3 million.[27] Since that time, the connection between employment and health insurance has strengthened, with the vast majority of working-age adults receiving coverage from their jobs. When President Truman proposed national health insurance in 1948, private insurance was already woven into the fabric of most people's lives and there seemed no urgency to bring about change. A new and powerful adversary had also joined the coalition against national health insurance—the insurance industry itself—which had a strong economic interest in maintaining the status quo. Over the last half-century, the benefits negotiated by the unions with their employers spread to all private insurance plans. In 1960, consumers paid out-of-pocket for 48 percent of all health care expenses, but only 15 percent in 2000 despite the ballooning costs of care. (This percentage has subsequently risen due to cost-shifting from employers to employees.) Two-thirds of Americans below age sixty-five were insured by employer-based plans.[28] Most citizens (i.e., those with insurance) saw no need to transform a failing system when the pain generated had no discernable effect upon them. However, for U.S. businesses such as the auto industry, and for those without health care coverage, it was different story.

Realizing that national health insurance was not an option during the 1960s because of opposition by the AMA and the health insurance industry, advocates concentrated on helping those segments of the population most in need: the elderly and the poor. They achieved their goals with the passage of Medicare and Medicaid in 1965, which gave vulnerable citizens health care coverage for both hospital care and physicians' services. Many believed this victory was merely a starting point and that national health insurance would be accomplished incrementally. But from that time on, even with Medicare to show as an obvious success, a program of government-run health insurance never received serious consideration in any reform proposals.

The next major change in the health insurance industry came with the wide-spread adoption of managed care with health maintenance organizations (HMOs). "Managed care is the enrollment of patients into a plan that makes cap-itated payments to health care providers on behalf of its members, thus shifting the financial risk for health care from patients to providers. The intent of this shift is to provide incentives to health care professionals to reduce their utiliza-tion of resources, ideally through measures such as health promotion and disease prevention among the group's members. The phrase 'managed care' is often used loosely to describe almost any attempt to limit health care expenditures in an increasingly competitive marketplace"[29] This method of delivering health care actually originated in the nineteenth century when physicians were prepaid by benevolent societies in urban areas to provide care for their members.[30] It was also seen in rural mining, lumber, and railroad towns, where workers and their families gave a fixed amount to physicians for care during a contracted period. But these arrangements did not gain much traction because of strong opposition by local and state medical societies.

During the Depression, however, the concept gained adherents as people across the nation were unable to afford basic care. A number of prepaid group practice plans were started, including the Group Health Association of Washington, D.C., the Group Health Cooperative of Puget Sound in Seattle, the Health Insurance Plan (HIP) in New York, and the Kaiser program on the West Coast, which was to become Kaiser Permanente. Though the governing struc-tures of these plans varied, they all offered affordable, comprehensive, prepaid care to their subscribers. Again, organized medicine, through the AMA, was vehemently against these plans and worked vigorously to abolish what they saw as a threat to physician autonomy, until the Supreme Court slapped them down for antitrust violations.

The San Joaquin County Medical Society in California in 1954 formed a med-ical foundation that collected capitation payments from enrollees and paid affil-iated physicians and hospitals for services on the basis of a relative value-based fee schedule.[31] This is believed to be an early prototype of the independent prac-tice association (IPA) model of prepaid health care. The group assessed quality of care, did peer review, and managed all the financial aspects of providing care.

As employer-based health care through insurance companies gave most young Americans coverage in the postwar years, followed by Medicare and Medicaid in 1965 for seniors, little thought was given to cost constraints. Patients were able to self-refer themselves to the legions of new specialists who used the latest expensive technology and treatments to provide care. Predictably, spending on health care skyrocketed, as patients bore little or no responsibility in paying for the services they utilized, and physicians were paid without scrutiny for every-thing they billed. In February 1971, the concept of HMOs and managed care received a big boost from President Richard Nixon, who pointed out the irra-tionality of the health care system then in place with its perverse incentives for providing services.[32] With 30 HMOs in operation at that time, Nixon wanted to generate 1,700 of them within five years, serving 40 million people, with a goal of covering 90 percent of Americans by 1980. What had once been decried by conservatives as utopian and socialistic, was suddenly seen by business and their Republican allies as a logical and efficient way to control costs. However, they also envisioned a change in structure and direction for these new organizations, from nonprofit or foundation-based to for-profit plans created and run by private health insurance companies. Legislation in 1973 appropriated $375 million to aid in the development of HMOs, while preempting state laws that prohibited pre-paid groups and mandating businesses with 25 or more employees to offer an HMO as one of their health care choices.[33]

From this governmental jumpstart, managed care became widespread in the United States over the next 25 years, even extending to Medicaid in some states. By 1999, managed care in various forms encompassed over half of the practicing physicians and more than three-quarters of the insured population.[34] The permutations included the traditional HMOs with salaried physicians; HMOs run by the insurance companies (with referrals to specialists required from primary care physicians and preapprovals necessary for major tests and many treatments); point of service plans (POS), which have more flexibility, but are more expensive; preferred provider organizations (PPOs), where subscribers are required to use the plan's network of physicians and hospitals whose fees are discounted; and the individual practice association (IPA) model, which is run by physicians. To hold down costs, many of these managed care plans relied on gatekeepers, either primary care physicians or administrators, to decide on the need for consultations, tests, and treatments.

Managed care was perceived by its proponents in the 1970s as a way to control the ever-escalating costs of health care and, for a brief period, appeared to be successful, at least in cutting the annual rate of increase. But by the late 1990s, the train of health care costs was back on track with yearly acceleration that was far in excess of growth in the nation's GDP. When analyzed carefully, the structure of the HMOs run by the insurance companies was not built to restrain costs. In fact, they started out at a cost disadvantage compared to nonprofit HMOs and programs such as Medicare. As described in Chapter 4, administrative overhead in the insurance company HMOs is 20–25 percent, and the high salaries of their executives (and their stock options), as well as profits for the stockholders, must be added to the direct costs of care. To be competitive and profitable, these companies have incentives to cut costs wherever possible, even if it impacts quality of care. Thus, we see the constant battles between the insurance companies and physicians over approval for tests and treatments, with patients fighting the companies because of a denial of services, sometimes even when they had been previously approved. The managed care companies have also forced an increase in physicians' overhead costs. New personnel had to be hired to interface over the telephone with insurance company staffs and file endless appeals for delayed or denied claims for services rendered. Managed care and the private insurance companies have not proven to be the solution to the problems of the health care system.

With about one-sixth of the population uninsured, states have been considering ways to help small businesses lessen the burden of obtaining health insurance for their employees.[35] These include granting tax credits to businesses that provide coverage for their workers and having the states create large pools of these companies to improve their purchasing power, while spreading the costs and risks. The insurance industry, however, has lobbied heavily against these pools, concerned that their profits would be reduced. Obstructionism by the insurance companies has consistently made health care reform measures more difficult to enact.

## The Pharmaceutical Industry

Apothecaries were found in most populous towns in Europe and the Islamic-world during medieval times. These were small businesses whose proprietors mixed herbs and other substances into compounds used to treat different ailments. The remedies that resulted were the product of local folklore, combined with the apothecary's imagination and resourcefulness, lacking any scientific basis for their supposed effectiveness. By the nineteenth century, these entrepreneurs began to be replaced by pharmaceutical companies that were able to manufacture drugs in large quantities. The local apothecary still created some compounds, while selling drugs made off the premises by the pharmaceutical firms (thus acting as a middleman). In time, large pharmaceutical companies were formed through mergers of the smaller ones or as the offspring of chemical companies and were able to dominate the marketplace. While some of their products may have had some medical value, many of these early companies sold patent medicines that were quite profitable, but provided no demonstrable benefit to patients. The landscape changed dramatically in the first third of the twentieth century, when scientific discoveries, such as insulin and penicillin, heralded the birth of the modern pharmaceutical industry.

As new drugs were developed, it became necessary to test them for safety and efficacy before the government would vet the drugs and allow them to be released for general public use. This process fell under the aegis of the Food and Drug Administration (FDA) and was long, arduous, and expensive. Patents on new drugs were granted for seventeen years, but much of this time could be consumed in testing and waiting for approval. The strength of the pharmaceutical companies lay not only in the approved drugs they were selling, but in those they had in the pipeline at various stages of development. Because of the huge expense of generating new drugs and bringing them to market, a number of the large drug companies also merged or were taken over by even larger competitors, often to gain control of their products. Many of the companies formed were multinational corporations able to market their medications all over the world. In the 1950s and 1960s, as many new drugs were created, the companies thrived. Among the new products were oral contraceptives, drugs to treat hypertension, various tranquilizers, and psychotropic medications. A host of other drugs followed to treat heart problems, diabetes, ulcers, epilepsy, and Parkinson's disease. The pharmaceutical companies with their huge profits became the darlings of Wall Street. This is no longer the case, however, due to the drug industry's own missteps, the lack of blockbuster drugs in the pipeline, and the possibility that health care reform will constrict their profits.

Public disenchantment with the drug companies has been fostered by the prices charged for patented drugs, which increases every year above and beyond the inflation rate. Companies with unique products that have patent protection can charge what they want for them and raise prices based on what they think the market will bear. This is irrespective of whether they have recouped their initial investments and made healthy profits and is unmoved by the financial pain they might cause patients. Medications in the United States are significantly more expensive than in other industrialized countries, with Americans subsidizing the cost of drugs elsewhere (discussed further in Chapter 4). The pharmaceutical industry maintains one of the most powerful lobbies in Washington, with huge campaign contributions to members of both political parties insuring that its voice will be heard. The drug companies and their lobbyists have pressured Congress not to enact laws that might interfere with their profits, and have even been able to get legislation passed that prohibits government agencies from negotiating lower prices with companies.[36] And just as the health insurance companies have done, pharmaceutical firms pay their top executives inordinately high salaries, as well as granting them stock options to insure more than generous total compensation. These expenses are supported by the high cost of prescription drugs and also impact the return to stockholders.

Another major problem currently for the pharmaceutical companies is the erosion of credibility that has occurred with both physicians and the public in relation to the safety and efficacy of their products. There are many examples that can be cited to show why this happened, but two stand out: Merck concealing the increased risk of heart attacks in patients taking the antiarthritis pain killer Vioxx and the ineffectiveness of Vytorin in preventing the buildup of plaque in the major arteries. Both of these were hidden from the public.

Vioxx is a nonsteroidal, antiinflammatory drug (Cox-2 inhibitor) that reduces the pain and swelling of arthritis. It was approved by the FDA in May 1999 and withdrawn by its manufacturer, Merck, in conjunction with the FDA, in September 2004.[37] It was pulled from the market after a study revealed an increased risk of heart attacks and strokes in patients on this medication. However, the heightened risk of these adverse events had been known since at least 2000, while the drug continued to be sold. Two million Americans were using Vioxx at the time it was removed, with over $2.5 billion in sales worldwide in 2003.[38] Though the FDA had required Merck to include warnings about possible cardiovascular events in the drug's information in 2000, the company had kept marketing Vioxx aggressively, both to physicians and the general public, while downplaying its risks. In addition to the negative publicity the Vioxx affair caused for Merck and the entire drug industry, the company has been sued by numerous patients who had heart attacks while they were on the drug. One reviewer for the FDA estimated in the medical journal *The Lancet* that possibly 140,000 heart attacks might have been caused by Vioxx before it was taken off the market.[39]

Vytorin, a blockbuster drug manufactured by Schering-Plough and Merck, contains two components, simvastatin (Zocor) and ezetimibe (Zetia), both of which lower cholesterol but by different mechanisms. On the market since 2004, it was expected that the two drugs in combination would be more effective than either alone in preventing heart attacks and strokes. However, a study released by the drug-makers in January 2008 revealed that the medication did not reduce the accumulation of plaque in patients' arteries, a precursor of heart attacks and strokes.[40] In fact, it was no more effective than simvastatin alone, a generic drug that was off patent. Though the results of this study had been available since April 2006, they were held back for more than a year and a half by the companies, during which time Vytorin had continued to be one of the world's best-selling drugs. It appeared that the medication was marketed to physicians and the public while the pharmaceutical companies were aware of its ineffectiveness, and that some of the data might have been manipulated to make the results seem better than they actually were.

Because of these two cases and other similar occurrences, claims from the pharmaceutical companies are now viewed with increased suspicion. Many physicians, as well as lay persons, believe the companies tend to pump-up the positive effects of their products, while not disclosing or minimizing negative data, with an indifference to patient safety in the pursuit of profits. Aggressive marketing to physicians of medications that are under patent protection is standard operating procedure, with their value denigrated when they become generic. (Drug companies spend more than $7 billion each year, about $10,000 per physician, in physician-directed marketing.[41]) In addition to advertising in medical journals and throwaways, drug representatives are a frequent presence in physicians' offices and hospitals, extolling the virtues of their firm's products. To capture physicians' attention, various small gifts used to be given away (pens, note pads, instruments, etc.), with office lunches and dinners at fine restaurants to promote particular medications. Though these would not seem to be significant enough to influence physicians' prescribing habits, they have been shown to generate a favorable bias, either consciously or unconsciously.[42] Recently, to avoid any possible conflicts of interest, a number of medical schools and hospitals have banned drug reps from their premises and prohibited their physicians from accepting gifts, free lunches, trips, or dinners.[43] (In July 2008, the pharmaceutical industry announced new guidelines that banned reminder gifts for prescription drugs such as pens, note pads, etc., but did not overhaul other incentives to physicians in any major way.[44])

Even more of a problem are so-called "consultants" for the drug companies—prominent physicians in practice or on the faculties of medical schools who are paid to advocate the use of company products. Depending on the financial arrangements, these "consultants" may be compensated to the tune of thousands to hundreds of thousands of dollars annually by the pharmaceutical firms, enough to crack any veneer of objectivity, with some physicians serving as consultants to several companies. (One Harvard child psychiatrist earned at least $1.6 million as a consultant to drug companies from 2000 to 2007, with another earning $1 million.[45] These physicians had promoted the use of certain psychiatric medications in children which benefited the companies through increased sales of their products.) Speakers bureaus are another method of rewarding physicians for endorsing drugs, with a fee given for short lectures or discussions (at a lunch or dinner) to other physicians about diseases that can be treated with a particular drug, or a talk about the drug itself. Unfortunately, many hospitals and teaching institutions, as well as medical associations, depend on money from the pharmaceutical companies to support their educational programs, again at a cost of compromising impartiality.

Direct-to-consumer advertising in all the media is also utilized by the drug companies to publicize their products, running the gamut from anticholesterol drugs such as Lipitor (and Vytorin), to migraine medications and therapies for erectile dysfunction and prostate enlargement. Celebrities, such as former Senator Bob Dole and artificial heart pioneer Robert Jarvik among others, have been used to endorse products.[46] Anyone who reads newspapers or magazines or watches television has undoubtedly encountered these advertisements, which exhort the reader or viewer to "ask your doctor about such and such." The marketing by the drug companies to physicians and the public costs billions of dollars, and while promoting various products, does nothing to enhance the quality of health care or make it more affordable. (In fact, it does the opposite.) If half the money these corporations spent on marketing was used instead to reduce the cost of their medications, it would be of great benefit to patients and society. (The pharmaceutical industry increased its spending for promoting its drugs from $11.4 billion in 1996 to $29.9 billion in 2005.[47] Direct-to-consumer advertising soared by 330 percent over this period, constituting 14 percent of the total.)

With some of the more important drugs aging and losing patent protection, they have been manufactured by generic drug companies both in the United States and abroad, cutting into the profits of the first-line pharmaceutical companies. To slow this process, the originators of the drugs have tried various legal maneuvers to tie up the generic companies, knowing that a delay of months or years can keep the prices high and bring in considerable income. In some instances, the first-line companies have also tried to buy off their generic competitors, making agreements (with payoffs) to keep the generics out of specific markets for a period of time to bolster their profits. There have also been efforts to promote studies by drug companies showing the superiority of their branded drugs to similar generic competitors, though the results of the studies have been questionable.[48] In addition, state legislatures have been lobbied in an attempt to prevent the insurers from switching to certain generic drugs.[49] (Unfortunately, the generic drug companies themselves often keep the prices of their products relatively high, knowing they are competing with even higher priced brand-name drugs. Thus, the savings to consumers and third-party payers may not be as great as they should be.)

In recent years, the pharmaceutical companies have been coming up with fewer blockbuster drugs than in the past. There seems to be less innovation from these companies as they have focused more on developing new variations of previously successful drugs, rather than finding completely new classes of compounds. This has constricted their profits and made it more critical for them to keep the prices of their existing products high and fight encroachment by the generic companies. Much of the innovation in terms of new therapeutic agents has been coming, instead, from biopharmaceutical firms of fairly recent vintage, such as Genentech, Chiron, and Amgen, among others. Biopharmaceutical agents are mainly protein compounds produced in cell cultures or animals through bioengineering, rather than combining chemical substances the way drugs were previously manufactured. Many of these agents are found normally in the human body and in larger amounts may moderate disease processes. They are extremely expensive and have greatly raised the cost of treatment for various medical conditions, while transforming many of the biopharmaceutical companies into success stories. (The use of these compounds and their cost will be discussed further in Chapter 4.)

## The Medical Device Industry

The medical device industry consists of a number of companies that manufacture devices, equipment, and appliances used to treat disparate medical conditions. Among the myriad of apparatuses being marketed by these corporations are stents, to open and maintain blood vessels; cardiac pacemakers and defibrillators; mechanical cardiac valve replacements and porcine valves (from pigs); bands to constrict the stomach in bariatric surgery; deep brain stimulators to treat Parkinson's disease and other neurologic conditions; artificial spinal discs and other hardware for spine surgery; artificial hips, knees, and other joints; dorsal column stimulators of the spinal cord to alleviate pain; shunts for hydrocephalus; and artificial limbs. Medical equipment companies that produce canes, walkers, hearing aides, and so forth, can also be considered part of this industry. Many of these companies are quite profitable, with their own coterie of lobbyists in Washington defending their interests from lawmakers and regulatory agencies. The major government division that regulates and monitors the use of medical devices is the Food and Drug Administration (FDA) through its Center for Devices and Radiological Health (CDRH). Unfortunately, the process of oversight is not as stringent as would be expected, with funding and personnel inadequate to the task. Some devices that have passed review have later been found to be unsafe, causing damage and death in patients. In fact, according to Consumers Union, 1.3 million Americans are injured each year by medical devices that have malfunctioned.[50] Over 450,000 emergency room visits in 2006 were caused by problems with medical devices, with 58,000 people dying at the hospital or requiring hospitalization.[51]

The same environment encountered at the drug companies raises questions about the medical device companies, including overpaid executives who are pressured to generate profits, inadequate concern for efficacy and patient safety, exaggerated claims of benefits, utilization of physicians to market products in disregard of conflicts of interest, and vigorous lobbying to achieve profitable ends. Though both pharmaceutical and medical device companies mouth the mantra of free markets and competition, they want it to apply only when they will benefit. And they are both willing to use political influence to fight competition when it may hurt their profits. A prime example of this is how Medicare purchases walkers for disabled patients. Congress has been setting the prices for medical equipment since 1989 and has Medicare pay $110 for a particular walker that can be bought at Wal-Mart for $60.[52] When Medicare decided to put different medical products out to bid to get the best prices, there was an outcry from the medical equipment makers, who began lobbying Congress and increasing their political contributions. In response, the House passed a law delaying the new policy, which was awaiting Senate scrutiny at the beginning of July 2008. This type of action highlights the systemic flaws in the health care system that need to be addressed as part of comprehensive reform.

## CHAPTER 4

# PROBLEMS WITH THE CURRENT HEALTH CARE SYSTEM

Much here does seem to be arranged in such a way as to frighten people off, and when one is newly arrived here, the obstacles do appear to be completely insurmountable.

—Franz Kafka, *The Castle*[1]

There are a number of major problems plaguing the U.S. health care system that must be addressed in any attempt at reform. Cost, complexity, and lack of access to care are three of the most important. Other problems for which solutions are needed include the linkage of coverage to employment, the shortage of primary care physicians, the variable quality of care, and medical negligence.

## Cost—Why Is U.S. Health Care So Expensive?

With the price of health insurance escalating yearly, many Americans today cannot afford the cost of coverage, and some of those with insurance have difficulty furnishing the co-pays and deductibles necessary to obtain medical care. Significantly, a recent government study found a wide and growing disparity in life expectancy between the wealthiest and poorest Americans.[2] Part of this may be related to lifestyle issues, but a large part is because of the cost of care. In confirmation, studies show that people who had no insurance had a marked improvement in their health when they enrolled in Medicare, particularly those who had diabetes or cardiovascular disease.[3] In my years of medical practice, I have seen individuals with serious ailments who did not fill prescriptions for some or all of their medications in spite of the possible consequences, because they did not have the means to do so. They were forced to choose which of their medications to buy and sometimes had to choose between medications and food. This is not an uncommon scenario. A Harvard study in Health Affairs in 2005 revealed that medical bills played a major role in about half of the nation's personal bankruptcies.[4] Over three-quarters of those who were financially devastated had health insurance at the beginning of their downward spiral. Illnesses, for some, led to the loss of their jobs and with it their insurance. Others simply could not manage the out-of-pocket expenses.

Besides the overall increase in health care spending, the portion for which the federal government is responsible (Medicare, Medicaid, the VA system, and various subsidies) is also rising rapidly, with a greater percentage of the budget devoted to health care than any other sector. A recent *New York Times* article noted that Medicare and Medicaid were responsible for nearly one-quarter of federal expenditures, $627 billion in the last fiscal year, with the expectation that this would double in the next decade.[5] Proposals by lawmakers to try and reduce disbursements in this area have not gained any traction, with the 2003 Medicare Drug Plan actually accelerating the anticipated growth.

Though there are many flaws in the dysfunctional U.S. health care system, the cost of care for individuals and society is seen by many as its single biggest

# Expenditures in the U.S.

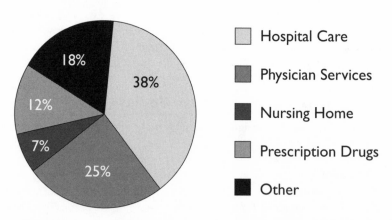

**Figure 4.1** Major areas where U.S. health care dollars are spent. Statistics for 2005 extrapolated to 2008—total health care spending of $2.1 trillion. (Other includes other professional services, home health care, non-prescription drugs, other medical durables and non-durables, vision products) Source: Center for Medicare and Medicaid Services, Office of the Actuary, National Health Statistics Group, National Health Expenditures Accounts.

problem. Health care spending since 1970 has increased annually at a rate of 9.8 percent, far above the expansion of the general economy as measured by the GDP.[6] Currently, over $2.1 trillion, costs are projected to reach $4 trillion in 2015, as previously noted. In 1970, health care accounted for 7.2 percent of U.S. GDP, rising to 16 percent in 2005, and anticipated to reach 20 percent by 2015. On a per capita basis, health care expenditures exploded from $356 in 1970 to $7,000 now, and are estimated to grow to $12,320 in 2015. Total costs will undoubtedly expand even further if health care reform is enacted without realistic constraints, as some or all of 46 million uninsured people suddenly enter the system.

If costs could be adequately controlled, other defects in the health care system could be confronted more aggressively. Coverage could be more easily provided for the uninsured. Enough physicians, nurses, and auxiliary medical personnel could be trained and hired to deliver services. There would be adequate supplies of vaccines, medications, and medical devices. Complex diagnostic testing would be available for everyone. Universal health care could be instituted and medical expenses would not bankrupt working families. In addition, U.S. businesses would not be handicapped by the vast sums they are required to spend on health care for employees and retirees. The federal government would also be able to devote more funding to priorities outside of health care and perhaps start paying down the national debt. There are many reasons why medical costs in the United States are currently so high and continue to increase. Some of the more important elements will be described.

### Demographic Factors

Demographic factors are one of the main drivers of U.S. health care costs. Though life expectancy is lower than in other developed nations, the number and percentage of older people is climbing, and will grow even further in the years ahead. In 2005, about 12 percent of the population was 65 or over.[7] By 2015, when more baby boomers reach age 65, this will rise to 14.5 percent. As the "boomers" move into their seventies and eighties, more than 20 percent of the population will be 65 or over, with 9 percent being 75 or over. Expensive, chronic illnesses are much more prevalent in older people. Seniors require far more hospitalizations, high-priced diagnostic tests, and costly treatments than the rest of the population, in addition to nursing home placement. Dementia alone currently affects 4 to 7 million people in this country, and that is projected to balloon to 14 million by mid-century. Just on the basis of an aging population, medical costs are headed through the roof if stringent reform measures are not instituted.

### Lifestyles

The unhealthy lifestyles of many Americans are another reason for mounting medical expenditures. More and more Americans of all ages are obese and do not exercise regularly, which leads to diabetes, hypertension, and elevated cholesterol. These features, in turn, contribute to more heart attacks and strokes, as well as a higher incidence of Alzheimer's and other forms of dementia, and a susceptibility to cancer. Extreme obesity increases the risk of diabetes seven-fold and hypertension six-fold, a recent report noted.[8] About 130 million people in the United States are either overweight or obese and over 9 million extremely obese.[9] Obese adults have nearly 40 percent higher health care costs than those of normal weight. It is estimated that 5–7 percent of the total, annual medical expenditures in the United States are the result of obesity. [10]

Independent of obesity, sedentary living is also a major risk factor for heart disease, strokes, dementia, and other grave illnesses. Yet, the vast majority of Americans have not gotten the message and refuse to exercise regularly. The Institute of Medicine, the medical division of the National Academies, advises at least an hour of exercise for everyone, every day, but very few Americans come close to following this guideline.[11] Unless there is a dramatic change in attitude, succeeding generations will continue to neglect physical activity, with the nation's children even now glued to television sets and video games, instead of running and playing. Many schools have also eliminated recess to provide more time for study, which is very shortsighted.

Cigarette smoking is another lifestyle choice that takes a heavy toll on U.S. health and pocketbooks. Around 436,000 lives are lost each year due to smoking-related diseases, and approximately 8.6 million people in the United States have at least one serious illness linked to the use of cigarettes.[12] Smoking is responsible for over $167 billion each year in health care costs.[13] Currently, about 21 percent of adults are smokers, and smoking is the leading cause of preventable death in the country.[14] Lung cancer, emphysema, and chronic obstructive pulmonary disease (COPD) are all overwhelmingly the result of smoking. In addition, cigarettes are an important risk factor for coronary artery disease, strokes, peripheral arterial disease, and several other types of cancer. Though nicotine is highly addictive, many motivated individuals are able to quit smoking each year. Not starting is an even better decision.

Drug addiction, alcoholism, and gun violence are responsible for a host of significant illnesses and injuries. These activities extract a high cost from society, not only in providing health care, but from the loss of productivity, use of the criminal justice system, imprisonment, and physical, emotional, and social rehabilitation. The estimated health care costs for drug abuse in 2002 was $15.8 billion.[15] Ten years ago, the National Institute on Alcohol Abuse and Alcoholism calculated the direct medical expenditures for alcohol abuse at $26.3 billion.[16] (The costs have undoubtedly grown considerably since the time of these analyses.)

### New Technology

Advances in technology over the last several decades have revolutionized medical care, extending lives and improving their quality, but also heightening costs. Numerous new diagnostic tools, procedures, drugs, and medical devices have been developed, many of which are extremely expensive. The use of angioplasty, stenting, and new drugs reduced the mortality from heart attacks nearly in half from 1980 to 2000—from 345.2 to 186 per 100,000 persons.[17] But this comes with a price of $40,000 to $60,000 for the management of each uncomplicated heart attack and even more if there are problems.[18] With new treatments, physicians are able to keep many people alive longer despite chronic illnesses, such as diabetes, AIDS, kidney disease, COPD, and cancer. However, this also means they will be treated for longer periods with expensive therapies. According to some experts, new medical technology may be responsible for half or more of the long-term growth in health care expenditures.[19]

Spending for diagnostic imaging is increasing faster than any other portion of medical care, growing at annual rate of 9 percent and reaching $100 billion in 2005.[20] Diagnostic imaging includes computerized tomography (CT) scanners, magnetic resonance imaging (MRI) scanners, and positron emission tomography (PET) scanners, each with various permutations and combinations, as well as bone scanners, single-photon emission computerized tomography (SPECT) scanners, and so forth. The price of many of these advanced instruments runs between $1 to $3 million each. The annual cost of operating an MRI machine is approximately $800,000,[21] with a CT unit somewhat less, and a PET the same or somewhat more. There were 900,000 PET scans performed in 2004, with an estimate that there will be over 2 million in 2010.[22] The number of CT scans skyrocketed from 3 million yearly in 1980, to 67 million in 2006.[23] 13.5 million MRIs were done in 2001,[24] the number undoubtedly rising since then. Charges for a PET scan range from $2,000 to $6,000 depending on the type of test, CT scans from $500 to $1,000, MRIs generally from $800 to $1,200.

The different scanners and machines are not only operated by hospitals for their patients, but by private entities seeking profits. The latter may include groups of radiologists, various practitioners (orthopedists, neurosurgeons, neurologists, cardiologists, etc.), and nonmedical corporations who hire physicians to read the scans. The underlying mantra behind these enterprises is a line from the movie *The Field of Dreams*: "Build it and they will come"—meaning that if a facility is erected, patients can be found to use it and generate income. A common practice for some of these corporations is to have the scanners in large vans, which are driven to different locations or different towns on a regular schedule if an area does not have enough patients to (profitably) support a full-time unit. An obvious conflict of interest arises when physicians are stockholders or owners of these expensive machines and refer people for the procedures. Given the price of these instruments and the high cost of running them, a steady stream of patients is necessary for the ventures to be profitable. This may lead to unnecessary tests being ordered, raising the costs of an individual's care and the cost to society.

Over the last several years, more than 1,000 cardiologists (and hospitals) have bought CT scanners for about $1 million dollars each to perform CT angiograms of the heart, charging their patients $1,000 or more per procedure.[25] These scans produce significant profits for the owners of the machines, but there is no hard evidence to date that the tests are beneficial for patients, and there could be an increased risk of cancer later on because of the radiation exposure.[26] Advertisements in all the media have been used to promote cardiac scans, with Oprah Winfrey and *Time* magazine praising them. In 2007, over 150,000 Americans had these scans at a cost of over $100 million. An article in the *New England Journal of Medicine* last year noted that "cardiac imaging has been increasing by 26 percent per year, despite a lack of evidence of outcome benefit."[27] Naturally, the cardiologists and radiologists who make money from these studies have been claiming they are helpful in diagnosing and treating patients, but there is a blatant conflict of interest here undermining their credibility. Though Medicare initially refused to pay for these tests, they relented after heavy lobbying by cardiologists, with private insurance companies following Medicare's lead. Paying for unproven, expensive technology is not the way to constrain health care costs.

Proton beam accelerators, used to treat prostate cancer and some other rare tumors, are the world's most expensive medical machines, priced at more than $100 million.[28] There are currently five of these therapy centers in the United States, with plans announced for over a dozen more and additional ones being considered. Though proton therapy can be beneficial in treating some very uncommon cancers, its value over traditional radiotherapy for prostate cancer is questionable. Yet, Medicare pays twice as much for this treatment ($50,000). Here again, proponents often have conflicts of interest. The huge expense for these machines in an era of exploding health care costs makes one wonder about the sanity of the entire system.

The last two decades have also seen an explosion in new types of treatments for many illnesses with a variety of pharmaceutical agents and a host of biopharmaceuticals. Medications, such as the statins to lower cholesterol and proton-pump inhibitors to treat gastroesophageal reflux disease and ulcers, are extremely effective, but quite expensive under patent protection. For example, Lipitor, a statin, which is the world's best selling drug, brought Pfizer $13 billion in annual sales at its height in 2006 (prior to another statin, Zocor, becoming available as a generic).[29] Each pill, from 10 to 80 mg, was sold at prices ranging from about 50 cents to $2.50 or more, depending on the quantity purchased and the venue where it was sold. One can imagine the cost of maintenance for patients who take these pills daily, even when they are insured and responsible only for deductibles and co-pays. The price of medications for other chronic conditions is similarly high, a drain on individual finances and government programs. Specialty drugs, such as Zofran, which is used to treat nausea from cancer chemotherapy, can cost from $10 to $20 for each pill.

A recent report by Express Scripts, one of the largest drug-benefit companies in the country, showed a sharp rise from 2000 to 2006 in the number of insured Americans who took prescription drugs.[30] It was observed that increased utilization of medications for diabetes, high blood pressure, cholesterol, GI problems, and depression elevated costs by 50 percent, or $12 billion. Significant geographical differences were noted, with states having the highest incidence of obesity using the most drugs.

The biopharmaceuticals, medications not even available 20 years ago, and developed by corporations of fairly recent vintage, including Amgen, Chiron, and Genentech, among others, now play an increasing role as therapy for a number of diseases. The treatment of multiple sclerosis and other autoimmune diseases, such as rheumatoid arthritis and ulcerative colitis, has improved dramatically with the use of these compounds, particularly some of the interferons and monoclonal antibodies. They are injected into the body subcutaneously or intramuscularly, or given through an intravenous infusion. Certain cancers may also respond to this type of therapy. These compounds, for the most part, do not cure the diseases they are targeting, but merely keep them under control. This means affected individuals will have to stay on these medications for the rest of their lives. And the cost of maintenance is astronomical. As an illustration, interferon therapy for multiple sclerosis runs between $25,000 to $30,000 per year, with similar costs for other diseases. Some monoclonal antibodies cost $4,000 to $8,000 for each treatment, and patients may receive them multiple times. Immune gamma globulin is in a comparable price range.

Two compounds highlight the problems of cost with some of the new therapies. One of these is Cerezyme, which is used to treat Gaucher's disease, a rare affliction that damages bone marrow, the liver, and spleen.[31] Cerezyme replaces an enzyme deficient in Gaucher's and arrests the deterioration. Only about 1,500 patients in the United States, and about 5,000 worldwide, take this medication. Because one company, Genzyme, has a monopoly on its production, the cost of Cerezyme tops $300,000 yearly for many patients.[32] Recently, controversy has arisen about the proper dose of the drug. Lowering the amount given could save individuals, insurance companies, and the government several hundred thousand dollars annually per patient. Although some researchers claim that smaller doses would be just as effective, the company has insisted that the full dose is necessary. (In 2007, Genzyme sold $1.1 billion worth of Cerezyme.)

A second biopharmaceutical raising questions about usage and cost is Avastin, a monoclonal antibody manufactured by Genentech, which inhibits a vascular growth factor and has been shown to be effective in some lung and colorectal cancers.[33] Recently, Avastin was approved for use in advanced breast cancer by the FDA after a scientific advisory committee had voted against it.[34] Though it temporarily halted progression of some of these cancers, a study did not show prolonged life when Avastin was used in combination with standard therapy. This was important because of severe side effects in some patients and the expense of treatment. For breast cancer, Avastin costs $7,700 per month or $92,000 annually. Median survival with the medication was 26.5 months, versus 24.8 months for those with standard therapy alone, less than two months difference. (The British National Health Service has not approved of its use in breast cancer, believing that the science did not justify its cost.) Even in lung cancer, when Avastin was given with standard chemotherapy, survival went from 10.2 months to only 12.5 months at a cost of $50,000 plus each year. (In the treatment of some cancers, cost can run up to $100,000 yearly.[35] Sales of

Avastin were about $3.5 billion last year, with the United States accounting for $2.3 billion. A number of other medications, particularly biopharmaceuticals, present similar dilemmas in terms of cost/benefit ratios.)

Avastin has also been shown to be of value in slowing progression in some cases of macular degeneration, when a small amount is injected into the eye in an off-label use of the medication.[36] However, Genentech has objected to it being employed in this fashion, as many ophthalmic patients can be treated with a single vial of the drug, lowering costs by a factor of 20 or more. Though this would make it more affordable to patients and save the government and insurance companies money, it would reduce profits for Genentech, which has a competing product on the market called Lucentis.

Recently, in an unprecedented move, Medicare agreed to cover cancer treatments with drugs that had not been approved by the FDA.[37] This occurred after intense lobbying by oncologists and cancer advocates to obtain payments for these off-label treatments of unproven benefit. Many of these biologic therapies are inordinately expensive, ranging in cost from $30,000 to $100,000 per year of treatment. They are generally utilized after all proven therapies have failed, providing false hope to severely ill patients at taxpayer expense.

### Medicare Part D and Drug Company Profits

Medicare Part D, to help seniors pay for prescription drugs, was passed by Congress in 2003 and has proven to be a windfall for the pharmaceutical companies. Offering moderate help to some older people, but of no benefit to many others, its complexity has been a major drawback to enrollees. As detailed by Congresswoman Louise Slaughter in a 2006 *New England Journal of Medicine* article, the bill was crafted by Republican legislators with the interests of the drug companies foremost, and a number of House rules were bent to line up the necessary support for passage.[38] The chairman of the House Commerce Committee who coauthored the bill, Billy Tauzin of Louisiana, was negotiating a job with a lobbying group for the drug industry (Pharmaceutical Research and Manufacturers of America [PhRMA]) that would pay him $2 million a year in salary, while the measure was before Congress. Then, following the bill's enactment, one of the top Republican aides on the committee resigned to also become a lobbyist with PhRMA. To ensure its passage, the Bush administration's Medicare chief, Thomas Scully, purposely low-balled the cost of the program and threatened to fire Medicare's actuary who wanted to release more accurate projections. (Scully left soon afterwards to take a job as a lobbyist for the health insurance industry.) It was estimated by independent analysts that the bill would boost drug company profits over the next eight years by $139 billion,[39] and, indeed, profits at these firms surged immediately after passage.[40] (When enhanced coverage for drugs under Medicare became available, pharmaceutical makers hiked prices sharply in the first quarter of 2006 to maximize their profits.[41]) Funding Medicare Part D will require a major increase in federal spending, as the government's share of prescription drug costs soared from

2 percent in 2005 to 27 percent in 2006.[42] Two of the more egregious aspects of the bill (and there were a number of them) prohibited Medicare from negotiating with drug companies for lower prices and banned importation of cheaper drugs from Canada, injuring both U.S. consumers and taxpayers, while helping the drug makers.

The pattern of maximizing profits irrespective of the impact on patients and society (as well as playing down adverse effects and questions of efficacy) are not unusual for the pharmaceutical and biopharmaceutical companies. One study in the 1990s noted that consumers in the United States paid 32 percent more for brand name drugs than in Canada and 60 percent more than in Great Britain.[43] Another study in 2003 showed that of the G8 industrialized nations, the United States was second only to Japan in prices for drugs under patent.[44] The six other countries paid 24–39 percent less than the United States for these drugs. (The United States did do better on prices for generics.) Another reason U.S. drug costs were so high was that its citizens utilized more of the newest, most expensive drugs, thus having by far the highest per capita drug expenditures of any nation.

### Characteristics of U.S. Medical Services

A recent report to Congress showed that the United States had far fewer doctor visits per person and fewer hospitalizations annually than other industrialized countries.[45] However, the intensity of diagnostic and therapeutic services was the highest, with more expensive, invasive procedures performed, along with a greater utilization of the newest technology. Hospital stays were also more costly, even though they were generally shorter in duration than elsewhere. As an example, an analysis of total hip repairs in Canada and the United States in 2004 found that the price in the United States was twice what it was in Canada, both for direct costs and overhead: $13,339 versus $6,766. Virtually all procedures and operations in the United States are more expensive than in other countries, with physicians' incomes also higher. Some U.S. businesses are even trying to reduce health care costs by sending employees to India for elective surgery, where medical costs are about 80 percent lower in first-rate hospitals with Western-trained physicians.[46] (Many hospitals in the United States are now having some of their x-rays, CT scans, and other imaging read by radiologists in India, both to save money and to have emergency coverage at night and on weekends.)

### Medical Advertising

Advertising by pharmaceutical companies, device makers, doctors, and health care facilities is also responsible for raising medical costs. Media ads hyping new diagnostic tests or treatments influence patients to ask their physicians for tests or medications that otherwise might not have been considered. Some physicians comply with these requests for fear of losing their patients if they refuse. In many cases, the new brandname medications that were lauded in the ads are no more effective than older drugs, but have more cachet because of the advertisements (and of course they are more expensive and profitable for the pharmaceutical firms). Occasionally, these newer medications also have adverse effects that have not been recognized. (Such was the case with Vioxx, the anti-inflammatory drug that increased the risk of heart attacks and was eventually withdrawn from the market.)

Though advertisements for screening CT scans tout their ability to pick up early cancers (or heart disease), the technique has not yet been proven to be of benefit. In addition, benign nodules or spots may be found that require biopsy or surgery to determine the cause, increasing the risk to patients and raising health care costs. One medical device maker, the Cordis Corporation, advertised its Cypher coronary artery stent directly to consumers during an National Football League football game on Thanksgiving Day, 2007, with the Medtronic Corporation having marketed its heart defibrillator to consumers previously.[47] Direct-to-consumer advertising for medical devices, such as artificial joints and heart stents, was estimated at $193 million in 2007.[48] Though it is difficult for consumers to judge the necessity for advertised tests and the value of suggested treatments, it is hoped by the corporate sponsors that patients will discuss the products with their doctors, who will then be more inclined to recommend them.

Physicians sometimes advertise having special skills or special equipment to deal with various conditions, particularly problems that may be refractory to therapy such as chronic fatigue syndrome, fibromyalgia, and low back pain. Desperate patients who have been frustrated by their inability to be cured or find relief may flock to these practitioners, who may be good at marketing, but don't have any unique expertise. In some cases, patients may be subjected to expensive diagnostic tests and treatments of questionable value by these doctors. And patients who have new problems and are attracted by these ads may have their diagnoses delayed because correct evaluation is not forthcoming. (Advertisements for procedures that are not medically necessary, not covered by insurance, and paid for out-of-pocket, such as cosmetic surgery, Botox, and Lasik eye surgery, can be regarded as independent of the health care system.)

### Internet Information

Patients' ability to gather medical information on the Internet has been a mixed blessing, enhancing knowledge in some cases, but producing anxiety and raising costs. A study by the Pew Research Center found that 80 percent of Internet users mine the Internet for health care guidance.[49] The sites utilized include WebMD, CDC Health Topics, DrKoop.com and a host of others that have been developed by physicians, medical schools, and government entities, as well as many for-profit enterprises, advocacy groups, and bogus experts. The problem is similar to that resulting from advertising, in that the information obtained is not always vetted and patients may interpret it improperly, proceeding to ask for tests and treatment that are not warranted. On the plus side, patients may learn more about their illnesses and ask pointed, intelligent questions of physicians. In this way, they may gain more understanding of their diseases and the different treatments available. However, patients may also focus on symptoms and diseases described on the Internet and self-diagnose, reinforcing hypochondriasis and causing needless stress. In addition, the Internet is a source where one can find alternative remedies, with extravagant claims made promoting drugs that may be of no benefit and some that are potentially harmful. These therapies may delay appropriate treatments with negative consequences.

## Unrealistic Expectations

Unrealistic expectations by patients also contribute to higher medical costs. Because of television programs that venerate physicians, newspaper and magazine articles extolling medical progress, and advances in technology, along with the ads from drug companies, device makers, and hospitals, many patients believe that an explanation can be found for all medical symptoms and that cures for virtually every ailment are possible. Unfortunately, this is often not the case, with causes of patients' symptoms remaining baffling after extensive work-ups and diseases that do not respond to treatment. However, some patients or their families are unwilling to accept diagnoses without hope and may demand expensive therapies that have no chance of success. If their physicians are unwilling to undertake treatment, the individuals or families may search for other doctors who are amenable to administering some sort of regimen, though the odds of breakthroughs are equally bleak. Sometimes this "doctor shopping" leads to consultations with multiple physicians until the patients or families find the answers they are looking for, whether valid or not. As long as Medicare or insurance companies are willing to pay for this kind of response and there is no financial disincentive for it, one can assume it will continue.

## Futile Care

Overlapping unrealistic expectations is the issue of futile care, a minefield at the borderland between ethics and cost. Some Americans believe every effort from a medical standpoint should be made to keep people alive, ignoring their prognoses and the extreme improbability of recovery. For a few, this even includes patients who are brain dead or infants who are neurologically devastated with no chance of significant improvement. The cost of caring for these unfortunate individuals, usually in the ICU on life-support machines, can be enormous. Futile care has a number of definitions, but basically it refers to medical intervention that does not have a reasonable chance of prolonging or saving a patient's life or restoring him or her to a decent quality of life. The ability to quantify this is difficult, with many subjective aspects and areas of conflict. Is it worthwhile resuscitating someone with terminal cancer or severe dementia, or treating his or her pneumonia? Should a person be kept alive on a ventilator in a vegetative state? Doctors and families vary in their approaches to these problems.

There is also an issue about providing kidney dialysis to patients with severe brain damage who have no chance of restoration of function. Currently, everyone who needs this treatment can receive it, no matter what their underlying status may be. Three hundred thousand patients a year are now on dialysis, at a cost of $16 billion, which is covered by Medicare.[50] A study published in 2006 revealed that 73 percent of dialysis patients had significant cognitive impairment.[51] Yet, if the patients or families want dialysis continued, it is.

As with unrealistic expectations, because third parties usually pay the bills for most of these patients, there may be no financial pressure for families to discontinue treatments. It is hard to legislate a universal way of dealing with futile care, and case-by-case considerations may continue to be necessary in the future.

### End-of-Life Care

End-of-life care in general is a significant driver of medical costs, with about 27 percent of Medicare's annual budget consumed by patients in their last year.[52] Much of this occurs in the last several weeks when patients are hospitalized. However, there are great regional variations in treatments and costs, including doctor's visits and hospitalizations. The average cost of the last six months of life in Manhattan in 2005 (the most expensive region) was $35,838, whereas in Wichita Falls, Texas (the least expensive) it was $10,913. Expense seemed to correlate with the number of physicians and hospital beds in a region, with more doctors meaning more (and more expensive) care. However, there are also great disparities in costs among major university hospitals, with Medicare spending for the last two years of life on average about $94,000 for those receiving most of their care at the UCLA Medical Center, compared to $53,000 at the Mayo Clinic, with other centers in between.[53] The differences were pronounced as well in the last six months of life, with about $53,000 at UCLA versus $29,000 at Mayo.[54] The tremendous ranges in cost may be a clue to savings if the question can be answered as to whether more expensive care extends life or improves its quality. Encouraging patients to have a living will and advanced directives would be helpful in saving money and resources for society and families, while making it more likely that they would die with dignity in the manner they wished.

(Over the last decade, physicians have been more aggressive in providing patients in their 90s, and even centenarians, with therapeutic interventions to prolong their lives.[55] Some of these invasive procedures would not have been done previously because of the associated risks. Though there are successes in this type of approach, it remains a matter of some controversy, both because of the costs involved and on a moral basis.)

### Malpractice and Medical Negligence

Malpractice and medical negligence increase health care costs, necessitating longer or new hospitalizations, additional tests or procedures, and even surgery, all of which can be expensive. Resolving liability and compensation for malpractice through the court system is an expensive process which is excessively prolonged and often does not deliver justice for either involved patients or physicians. To try and protect themselves, doctors purchase malpractice insurance, which runs from thousands to hundreds of thousands of dollars annually, depending on the medical specialty and risk, previous actions against the doctor, and the state environment for lawsuits. The cost of this is recouped in the fees charged to patients. An article 20 years ago in the *Journal of the American Medical Association* estimated that the cost of medical liability insurance was responsible for "approximately 15 percent of the total expenditures on physicians' services."[56] It has most likely risen since then, given the ballooning costs for this insurance.

Practicing defensive medicine is seen by physicians as a bulwark against malpractice suits, but it heightens health care costs, as well as occasionally causing pain and suffering for patients. By defensive medicine is meant the ordering of tests and procedures of limited value to protect doctors in the event of lawsuits. It can lead to unnecessary consultations with specialists, unnecessary surgery, and unnecessary Caesarian sections, all of which are expensive. The burden defensive medicine places on the health care system is difficult to assess, particularly as much of this behavior has become ingrained in physicians. Estimates in 2005 ranged from about 1 percent of health care costs, $20 billion, up to $60–$108 billion.[57] (Medical negligence and malpractice are major health care problems independent of their effect on cost and will be discussed further in the following chapter.)

### Overhead, Administrative Expenses, and Waste

Overhead, administrative expenses, and waste take a major bite out of Americans' health care dollar. One study found that of health care spending in 2003, at least $399 billion went to overhead and administration, or 24 percent.[58] (Over 27 percent of health care employees were utilized in administrative functions.) Other articles have mentioned administrative costs in the range of 15–25 percent.[59,60] On the other hand, Medicare's administrative costs are about 2–3 percent, with similarly low expenses for the European health care systems.[61] If 20 percent is used as the figure for health care overhead in the United States, with current total expenditures of $2.1 trillion, $420 billion of that is consumed by administrative costs. (Any program of health care reform that cut overhead in half would save $210 billion dollars a year, the annual savings increasing as spending continued to rise.)

Waste occurs mainly through duplication of services. Though its cost is difficult to assess, it is likely to be considerable. With patients often seeing different specialists for various problems and having tests and procedures done in different settings, studies may be unknowingly repeated. At times, medications may also be prescribed or treatments given that have previously been tried unsuccessfully and are employed again because the information was unavailable. (Aside from cost, there is the potential danger of adverse effects.) Electronic health records (EHRs) are supposed to reduce the duplication of services, but until the utilization of

EHRs is more widespread, with greater access by all practitioners and with standards in place for inter-operability, this type of waste will continue unhindered.

### Fraud

Because of the complexity of the health care system, fraud is a continuing problem that is estimated to extract between $54 and $100 billion in funds each year.[62,63] In the year 2000, the Department of Justice negotiated or won over $1.2 billion in health care fraud cases.[64] Though there were 457 criminal indictments awaiting resolution and 467 convictions, along with 233 civil cases filed and nearly 2,000 pending, they were only a small piece of the total picture. Fraud can be committed by large corporate entities or by individual practitioners, the most frequent offenses being billing for services not performed, overbilling, upcoding for various services, and illegal kickbacks.

The Department of Justice in December of 2004 ended a longstanding case with Hospital Corporation of America after the company pleaded guilty to criminal conduct and finalized a settlement of $1.7 billion with the government.[65] (HCA is an enterprise of the Frist family, with Bill Frist, the former Senate Republican majority leader from Tennessee, his father, and brother all deriving their fortunes from the company.) The settlement acknowledged false claims to Medicare and other federal programs, kickbacks to physicians, and other unlawful practices. Another case in 2004 against Gambro Healthcare, a dialysis company, brought the government $350 million in criminal fines and penalties and over $310 million to resolve civil liabilities.[66] The company was cited for kickbacks to physicians, false statements to obtain payment for unnecessary tests and services, and payments to a sham company. Recently, medical supply companies were cited by Congressional investigators for having defrauded Medicare of tens of millions of dollars by using ID numbers of dead physicians to obtain payments for the apparent use of various kinds of medical equipment.[67] Some of these physicians were still listed as active Medicare providers, though they had died ten or fifteen years earlier.

In spite of the examples of corporate fraud brought to the attention of the media and the public, even more cases by both large businesses and individual practitioners never see the light of day. Billing for unsubstantiated services and upcoding are common practices for some physicians and other health care providers. (For example, a dermatologist may bill for a three-minute removal of a tiny skin lesion for $500 to $1,000 as a surgical procedure. Or, a urologist may bill $250 for a bladder ultrasound that takes less than five minutes on every follow-up visit in order to boost reimbursement, even if it is not medically indicated.) Most of the success of these schemes is due to lack of oversight and negligence by the insurance companies and governmental authorities, who are willing to pass the costs on to consumers and taxpayers. Though careful scrutiny by sophisticated computer programs and forensic accountants of medical bills and the overall pattern of charges would help to detect fraud, whistle-blowers given the promise of monetary rewards more often provide a direct route to the perpetrators. (In 2008, Medicare began a new program of auditing physician and hospital claims, searching for overpayments from inaccurate coding.[68]) On the other hand, insurance companies often cut payments to physicians for their services unilaterally and deny or delay reimbursement.

### Unnecessary Medical Care

Medically unnecessary and/or excessive care may be responsible for 20 to 30 percent of total health care spending in the United States according to the Center for Evaluative Clinical Sciences at Dartmouth Medical School.[69,70] If the high end of this estimate is valid, $630 billion is being squandered on care that does nothing to prolong or improve American lives, with at least $420 billion being wasted at the low end. (One Congressional Budget Office estimate places it at $700 billion.[71]) Included under this umbrella are extraneous office visits, useless procedures, superfluous treatments with drugs and medical devices, and unneeded hospitalizations. Indeed, some of this unnecessary care results in adverse outcomes that cause injuries (adding to medical costs) and even premature deaths.

The incentives for excessive care are built into the health care system itself, where conflict of interest is an integral part of the delivery of medical services. Remuneration for physicians and other providers is dependent on the volume of patients seen, the number of procedures done, and the amount and intensity of services performed. The gatekeepers who decide whether these services are warranted are usually the physicians themselves, who then arrange the procedures that they themselves carry out, schedule office visits, and recommend hospitalizations. For instance, cardiologists derive most of their income from diagnostic testing, catheterization studies, placing of stents, and other invasive and noninvasive procedures, far exceeding consultations and time spent with patients. Similarly, gastroenterologists receive much greater compensation for doing endoscopies and colonoscopies than for seeing patients. Surgeons are paid primarily for the operations and procedures they perform that they themselves are expected to recommend or reject. Primary care physicians often generate a large proportion of their income from simple laboratory tests done in their offices, such as blood work, x-rays, and EKGs. Even assuming that all physicians are highly ethical and only perform procedures they deem important, it would take saintly individuals not to be biased in favor of the decisions that provide them with financial rewards.

Among the most common unnecessary procedures are hysterectomies (removal of the uterus), spine surgery, knee arthroscopy (inserting a small flexible tube into the knee joint), and angioplasty (opening up clogged arteries with a balloon and usually placing an expandable mesh to keep the artery open, i.e., a stent). Hysterectomies are often recommended as the answer for uterine fibroids (benign tumors), but many of the 600,000 hysterectomies performed each year may not be needed.[72] Some of these patients require no procedure at all, whereas others can be treated by fibroid embolization, a nonsurgical alternative. But gynecological surgeons lose money each time they refer a patient for embolization instead of operating.

The Associated Press reported on an American College of Cardiology meeting in March of 2007, where it was suggested that over a half million angioplasties each year were unnecessary or premature out of 1.2 million that were done.[73] In a study published two weeks later in the *New England Journal of Medicine* involving over 2,200 patients, it was shown that those with stable coronary disease did just as well with medical treatment as they did with angioplasties.[74] Yet, in spite of studies that cast doubt on the need for all the angioplasties being done, many are still performed unnecessarily, benefiting the physicians who are intervening. Cardiologists realize $2,000–$5,000 for each angioplasty, but receive only a few hundred dollars for treating patients with medication. (About one-third of patients who initially receive medication may eventually require angioplasty or coronary bypass.)

MRIs of the knee joint may now provide information that previously could only be obtained by arthroscopy, a procedure performed by orthopedists. Though this operation is also done to remove torn cartilage, it was estimated in one report that 33 percent of arthroscopies were unnecessary.[75]

Spinal operations are commonly utilized to remove herniated disks, correct boney arthritic changes that press on the nerve roots, and to stabilize the spine. However, studies have shown that lumbar disks can regress over time without surgery, and that surgical and nonsurgical disk patients improve comparably over a two-year period.[76] This is an obvious argument for conservative treatment of patients with herniated disks, though the neurosurgeons and orthopedists who perform the surgery lose considerable sums for each operation they miss. The fact that there is a 15-fold geographical variation in the number of diskectomies performed in the United States, and a lower ratio internationally, also suggests that many of the U.S. operations are inappropriate.

Spinal fusion surgery increased 77 percent in the United States from 1996 to 2001 after the FDA approved the use of special devices to aid the fusion.[77] An article in *The New England Journal of Medicine* in 2004 questioned the value of this type of surgery and whether it resulted in significant improvement in quality of life.[78] Among Medicare patients, the risk of complication was doubled in those who had spinal fusion compared to other spine surgery, as was postoperative mortality. Again, there was a wide regional variation in the use of this technique. The authors of the article wondered whether the increase in spinal fusion operations was due to financial incentives for the surgeons, hospitals, and medical device makers, rather than because of proven benefits. In addition to an average hospital bill of $34,000, professional fees exceeded $10,000–$15,000. (The number of spinal fusions performed annually in the United States climbed to 300,000 in 2008, at an average cost of $59,000.[79]) Spinal implants and devices were noted to be a $2 billion a year industry in 2004, with an 18–20 percent growth rate.[80]

Another example of how financial incentives for physicians affect behavior is evident in the prescribing patterns for anti-anemia drugs (Epogen, Aransep,

Procrit) for cancer and kidney dialysis patients. The higher the doses of these drugs, the more the pharmaceutical companies are reimbursed for them. Apparently, Amgen and Johnson and Johnson, two of the major drug companies, gave rebates to physicians on their drug purchases worth hundreds of millions of dollars, to get them to prescribe high doses of anti-anemia drugs to patients under their care.[81] Not only were these levels unnecessary, they also increased the risk of vascular complications in these patients, such as heart attacks or strokes. These payments from the drug companies are apparently legal and a major source of income for these physicians and their medical centers. (One group practice of six oncologists was given $2.7 million by Amgen in 2006 for prescribing $9 million worth of its drugs.)

At times, the line blurs between unnecessary care and outright fraud. In 2006, Tenet Healthcare agreed to pay $500 million to settle claims that physicians at Redding Hospital in California had performed unneeded surgery.[82] An unusually high number of coronary bypass operations per capita (two to three times the expected rate) had been done at the hospital which was owned by Tenet Healthcare. In another settlement as part of the case, Tenet assented to pay $900 million to Medicare and sell eleven hospitals to resolve charges of overbilling the government $1.5 billion.

Another aspect of unnecessary care is that there are some non–evidence-based treatments that may be lengthy and costly. A prime example of this is the therapy given by some doctors for chronic Lyme disease. The acute form of the disease is caused by a small organism (spirochete) spread by the bite of an infected tic. It causes a characteristic rash, joint pains, fever, and headaches and is effectively treated with a short course of oral antibiotics. However, a few patients develop chronic, nonspecific symptoms including fatigue, generalized aches and pains, problems with memory and concentration, and weakness. There are a small number of physicians who place these patients on long-term intravenous antibiotics, which are extremely expensive and have not been shown to be of any greater value than brief courses of oral antibiotics. Other costly therapies that have been given include intravenous immune globulin, again without proven benefits. Some patients say they subjectively feel better when receiving these treatments, but there is no evidence that they work. Other conditions may be managed in a similar fashion without supporting data.

### Insufficient Emphasis on Prevention

Health care costs are also increased because physicians are paid mainly to diagnose and treat diseases rather than to try and prevent them. They are not compensated adequately for discussions with patients about lifestyle issues, such as smoking, lack of exercise, diet, compliance with medication regimens, the dangers of alcohol and drug abuse, or for managing chronic illnesses. In fact, there are disincentives for this type of time-consuming activity. The volume of patients seen and in-house tests obtained determines the income of primary care physicians, not time spent talking to patients. And why should a cardiologist tackle diet and exercise with two patients for a half-hour each, when he can make 20 times as much doing a catheterization study. To benefit patients and lower costs, prevention and/or early treatment of chronic diseases, such as diabetes, hypertension, coronary artery disease, and chronic lung disease, makes much more sense than trying to control them afterwards with all the many expected complications. (Recently, there have been some experimental programs by insurance companies, state, and federal agencies to increase payments to primary care physicians and have them spend more time with their patients, hoping that this will result in cost savings later on.[83])

### Undocumented Immigrants and Uncompensated Care

Uncompensated care given to undocumented immigrants is a relatively minor factor in heightened health care costs. Though this care consumes only a small fraction of total national expenditures, it has overwhelmed some local facilities that treat large numbers of these immigrants, bankrupting the institutions and forcing them to close. A study by the Federation for Immigration Reform estimated that the cost of uncompensated health care for the 2.2 million undocumented immigrants in California in 2004 was $1.4 billion.[84] With 12–14 million of these immigrants in the country, that projects to approximately $8.5 billion spent nationally.

### Insurance Company Actions to Bolster Profits

Aside from administrative waste and overhead, insurance companies raise the cost of health care with unethical actions in their quest for profits. Though these profits may benefit stockholders, the main beneficiaries are the company executives who reap millions to hundreds of millions of dollars. An article in the Wall Street Journal in April of 2006 described how the CEO of UnitedHealthcare, William McGuire, made $8 million in salary plus bonuses and perks, and had accumulated $1.6 billion in unrealized gains in stock options.[85] The directors of the company had allowed McGuire to time his stock option grants when prices were low to enhance his profits and it appeared that he had backdated some of these options. The author observed how "an elite group of companies is getting rich from the nation's fraying health-care system. They're middlemen who process the paperwork, fill the pill bottles and otherwise connect the pieces of a $2 trillion industry. ...They're bringing in profits—and their executives are among the country's most richly paid—as doctors, patients, hospitals, and even drug makers are feeling a financial squeeze."[86] (It should be remembered that this description of the insurance companies came from the Wall Street Journal, the icon of capitalism.) It was also noted that Leonard Abramson, the founder of U.S. Healthcare pocketed $900 million in 1996 when he sold his company to Aetna. Most other CEOs and executives of health insurance companies have also been generously rewarded, while the price of coverage was skyrocketing and there are now 46 million uninsured. Ironically, UnitedHealth's mission statement includes—"improve access to health and well being services; simplify the health care experience; promote quality; and make health care more affordable."[87]

In starting the process and assessing potential policyholders, insurance companies attempt to insure only the healthiest patients, rejecting small groups or individuals with pre-existing conditions or those whose previous experiences suggest high utilization of medical services. Health insurance was originally envisioned to spread risk throughout a community so that those unfortunate individuals with serious illnesses could afford care and would not be unduly burdened financially. However, the insurance companies have subverted this concept to enhance their profits. "Cherry-picking" by the insurance companies has made it impossible for many people to obtain coverage and has increased the ranks of the uninsured. One group that has particular problems includes those who retire before age 65 when they can be covered by Medicare. Though the Consolidated Omnibus Budget Reconciliation Act (COBRA) allows individuals to purchase the insurance provided by their previous employers, coverage only extends for 18 months, after which they are on their own. The cost of individual health insurance policies makes it prohibitive for many Americans, even if they have no preexisting conditions.

In May 2008, after some of the major health plans announced disappointing earnings to Wall Street, they affirmed that they were willing to lose members (and increase the ranks of the uninsured) in order to protect their profit margins.[88] The president and CEO of Wellpoint told analysts: "We will not sacrifice profitability for membership."[89] Small businesses have been particularly hard hit by the increase in health insurance costs, with many simply dropping coverage. And because of consolidation among the major insurance firms, there is less competition, allowing companies to raise premiums for policyholders and put pressure on physicians to accept lower fees. There is no consideration about responsibility to the public because of the special role these companies play.

For those individuals who have managed to get insurance, health insurance companies, and health maintenance organizations (HMO) have further structured the system to maximize their profits, placing barriers in the way of patient approval for various diagnostic studies and treatments, many of which are fairly routine. Often, there are long waits to get through to their panels for the required phone request and explanation. Then, if approval is granted, the companies may later renege or delay payment, leading to additional fighting with the company by patients or providers. Another scheme is to pay providers at lower than agreed rates for services, forcing providers to argue with the companies or bill patients for the underpayments. In January 2008, United Health Group and several of its subsidiaries were charged by New York's attorney general Andrew Cuomo, "with defrauding consumers by manipulating reimbursement rates for patient visits to out-of-network doctors."[90] By lowering what was considered reasonable and customary rates for physician services, they were able to decrease their reimbursement to these physicians (80 percent of reasonable and customary), obligating the patients to pay more. This type of invidious behavior by health insurance companies, with numerous other repugnant strategies, is common place and has been experienced repeatedly by participating physicians and patients.

Another recent change by the insurance companies to enhance profits is their institution of a Tier 4 level in their drug reimbursement plans,[91] and even a Tier 5, both of which involve cost-sharing by patients for special drugs.[92] Previously, patients paid a fixed amount for each prescription (e.g., a co-pay of $20) that was independent of the cost of the medication. With Tier 4, the insurance companies are charging patients a percentage of the cost of the most expensive drugs, anywhere from one-fifth to one-third. This can mean hundreds to thousands of dollars a month, which patients with illnesses like cancer, multiple sclerosis, and rheumatoid arthritis have to pay in order to be treated. Many of these seriously ill patients can not afford the cost of these drugs and may have to discontinue therapy. This is yet another action by the insurance companies that runs counter to the basic reason health insurance came into being in the first place—to spread risk around a large group of subscribers to pay for the care of those patients with high-cost illnesses and unusual medical expenses. (The question must be asked whether these for-profit companies that are trying to bolster their bottom lines in every way possible can play a constructive role in health care reform, where patients' needs should come first.)

Some of the elements responsible for the high cost of health care in the United States are beyond the control of the government or corporate entities, such as

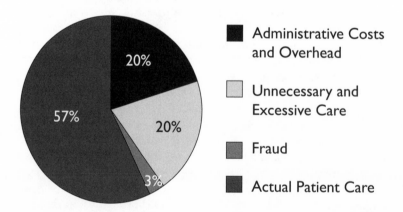

**Figure 4.2** Percentage of health care spending that goes to patient care. Source: Center for Medicare and Medicaid Services, Office of the Actuary, National Health Statistics Group, National Health Expenditures Accounts.

people living longer and having more chronic illnesses as they age. Other areas, such as unhealthy life styles, can possibly be reversed through education and/or incentives over decades. However, as has been shown, there are other factors in the health care equation that are ripe for aggressive intervention. These include bloated overhead, administrative costs, and waste (estimated to squander 15–25 percent of the nation's $2.1 trillion health care bill annually), unnecessary and excessive care (estimated to consume 20–30 percent), fraud (at $50 to $100 billion), and defensive medicine (at $20–$108 billion; this may fall under the heading of unnecessary care. All together, it appears that 40–50 percent of U.S. health care spending is dissipated in areas not directly related to care itself and which does nothing to improve or prolong people's lives. Reallocation of just a portion of this money could easily provide coverage to all of those without health insurance, could procure better care for those within the system, provide appropriate compensation to physicians for quality care, and pull Medicare away from its future financial abyss.

## Complexity

Although cost may be the elephant in the room in terms of shaping health care reform, there are other problems that must also be addressed. The complexity of the system is one of the most frustrating, with both patients and physicians having difficulty navigating the labyrinth of coverages, charges, co-pays, deductibles, and required approvals for various tests and treatments. Of course, this only occurs after a person has insurance and goes to see a physician or needs a medical service. Trying to analyze and choose an insurance plan in the first place can in itself be a daunting experience, with hundreds of companies and thousands of plans with multiple options offered in different markets within the United States. It did not start off this way. At the beginning of the last century, medical care involved a one on one exchange between doctor and patient, with direct payment for services that were generally reasonable. The increased frequency of more expensive hospital care and treatments led to the growth of health insurance during the 1920s and 1930s, exploding during and after World War II. Subsequently, health insurance for working adults and their families has been linked to employment, with seniors covered by Medicare, the impoverished by Medicaid, and one-sixth of the population uninsured.

Traditional insurance was known as indemnity, or fee for service, where the insurance company reimbursed the patient or paid the physician or hospital a portion of any charges. However, as costs began to accelerate without any constraints on fees, new kinds of insurance plans became dominant in the 1980s and 1990s in an attempt to bring costs under control. Under many of these "managed care" plans, fees for participating physicians were capped and prior approvals from the insurance companies were expected before expensive tests or treatments could be ordered. This required patients and physicians to become acquainted with the intricacies of these plans to be certain they were not being denied benefits. Contesting the decisions of the insurance companies was time consuming and filled with obstacles, which only the most tenacious could overcome, with constant battles for approval and reimbursement occupying patients and physicians' staffs. This is how it has remained to the present.

Ideally, patients should know which charges will be covered, what are reasonable and customary fees, what exclusions are part of the package, what are the maximum out-of-pocket expenditures, whether there is a cap on the total the company will pay for an illness (yearly, for a lifetime), how does drug coverage fit into the plan, how do preexisting conditions impact benefits, what is the value of catastrophic versus comprehensive coverage, and so forth. However, very few policyholders are aware of all the features of their policies until their company withholds payment for some service and they are forced to look at the fine print. Managed care of one sort or another now rules the insurance world, as patients deal with various forms of health maintenance organizations, preferred provider organizations, and point of service plans. Recently, health savings accounts have been introduced as a different approach to pay for medical care. There is also Medicare with its various supplemental plans and Medicaid. With some of the managed care plans, a primary care physician acts as a gatekeeper, referring patients to specialists when the conditions are beyond his or her comfort zone. But the ultimate decisions about what services will be paid for, and at what level, remain with the insurance companies.

As mentioned previously, the system that has evolved necessitates hordes of administrators for both providers and the insurance companies to joust over approval and benefits, greatly increasing overhead expenses. (Some primary care physicians refer patients to specialists so they themselves will not have to fight to get tests approved that they know are necessary.) The complexity also makes access to care more difficult for those with insurance, as they have to wait for approval for many services. It impacts quality of care as well, as delay at times can lead to bad outcomes and certainly raises the stress level of patients.

One of the goals of health care reform must be to reduce the unfathomability of the system, making it more user-friendly by requiring straight forward standard terms that would allow patients to understand the provisions of their coverage and help physicians to deliver the best care possible.

## The Uninsured

The lack of health care coverage for nearly one-sixth of the nation's population (46 million people), and the restrictions they face on access to care, is another major failing of the current system. Though a large proportion of this group is young and healthy, many others are older members of the working-poor whose children may be covered through government programs, such as State Children's Health Insurance Program (SCHIP). Without primary care physicians to monitor their health, the uninsured use hospital emergency rooms to treat acute illnesses and injuries, ignoring prevention, and control of chronic conditions.

With delays in diagnosis and treatment, the uninsured have higher rates of morbidity and mortality from common illnesses and a reduced life expectancy compared to the rest of Americans. (A recent study showed that patients who were uninsured or had Medicaid were more likely to be diagnosed with cancer in the late stages of the disease than those with private insurance, reducing their chances of survival.[93]) It may also ultimately cost more to treat their medical problems, and they may be less productive members of society because they are disabled or sick. In addition, caring for the uninsured raises health care costs for other citizens and causes financial difficulties for those hospitals with a large proportion of these patients.

Even middle-class Americans who have health insurance have experienced problems obtaining care recently, because they could not afford the high deductibles and co-pays that were part of their coverage. These "underinsured" grew to 25.2 million people in 2007, up from 15.6 million in 2003, as reported in a study from the Commonwealth Fund.[94] Being "underinsured," also delays the diagnosis and treatment of potentially serious illnesses, increasing both the social and economic costs.

The United States is the only developed nation that does not provide health care for all of its citizens. Universal, affordable access to care must be one of the pillars of any reform program.

## Linking Health Insurance to Employment and the Lack of Portability

The linkage between employment and health care coverage for working-age adults in the United States is another problem ingrained in the current system. After World War II, labor contracts between the unions and industry solidified this relationship, and it was accepted by the nation's citizens as the normal way that health insurance should be obtained. However, as costs for care escalated over time, providing health insurance for workers and retirees created a significant financial burden for U.S. industries, making the nation's products less competitive in the global economy. Aside from the handicap this connection to health care places on U.S. industry, it does not make sense for a number of other reasons.

For one, a large percentage of the working-age population is not employed by major corporations who are able to spread risk among numerous policyholders and negotiate the best costs with insurance companies, or even self-insure. Many workers labor for small businesses that have problems finding insurance at reasonable rates and may not offer coverage. It may be even more difficult to obtain insurance for professionals, those who are self-employed, and those who are temporarily out of work. And for the long-term unemployed, it is nearly impossible. The plans in force by businesses are also diverse, with some including family members with or without additional payments, covering children up to certain ages, having different co-pays and deductibles, and being responsible for different services. There is also the question of why employers should assume the costs of health care in perpetuity for individuals who once worked for them, covering retirees decades after they have left the workplace. The linkage of businesses to health care coverage certainly renders the system more complex and fragmented and does nothing to lower costs or improve the quality of care.

Another major failing of the current arrangement is that it ties employees to the businesses that provide them with health care even when they are unhappy with their jobs, wish to seek other opportunities, or go out on their own, for fear they will be unable to find affordable coverage. This lack of portability distorts the normal marketplace for labor and is a detriment to start-up companies, innovation, and entrepreneurship. A person's risk for illness does not change when he or she leaves a job, and there is no reason why employment should be a prerequisite for health insurance. Ending the connection between employment and health care with universal coverage should be a mainstay of any reform proposals.

Indeed, corporations in the United States appear to finally be backing reform and want to get out of the health care business. Unable to control its costs, they see it as a losing proposition that will further erode U.S. global competitiveness in the future, particularly since other nations have universal care. The Coalition to Advance Healthcare Reform was created in May 2007, by more than 50 employers and business leaders, to promote reform on both the federal and state levels.[95] In addition to other businessmen, these executives see the need for universal health care coverage and favor market-based solutions through government legislation. However, participation in this group by the CEOs of some of the major health insurance companies calling for a "public/private partnership that creates a market to offer affordable health care to all"[96] has to make one skeptical about the motivation of all the members. But in general, corporate executives are cognizant of the crisis in health care and the necessity for meaningful reform.

## The Shortage of Primary Care Physicians

There are a number of aspects to be considered regarding the shortage of primary care physicians and maldistribution in terms of the fields chosen by those entering the medical profession. Men and women select medicine as a career for various reasons. These include a compassionate nature and a desire to help people, the intellectual challenge that medicine presents, and the possibility of being involved in scientific breakthroughs. There is also a certain prestige associated with being a physician, with respect and admiration from the community, friends, and family. In addition, medicine in the past has meant earning a good living and being able to support a family in a comfortable style. This last statement is no longer completely true, as there is a great variation in earnings among different fields of medicine, with many practitioners currently struggling from a financial standpoint. This is exacerbated by the heavy indebtedness that doctors face after the years of undergraduate and medical school, internship, residencies, and fellowships, which can add up to hundreds of thousands of dollars, which must be paid off with interest. (In 2001, 23 percent of medical school graduates had debts of $200,000 or more.[97] Overall, 87 percent were indebted, the median amount being $145,000 for graduates of public medical schools and $180,000 for private medical school graduates.)

A Medical Economics survey of physician salaries in 2003 showed median compensation of all respondents to be $162,000, going from a low of $116,000 for general practitioners to $360,000 for invasive cardiologists.[98] Gastroenterologists and orthopedists were at $300,000, general surgeons at $230,000, internists at $150,000, and pediatricians at $130,000. However, a significant percentage of cardiologists, gastroenterologists, and orthopedists earned over $400,000 annually. A number of other high earning specialties, such as neurosurgery, ENT, cardiac surgery, radiology, dermatology, and anesthesia were not included in this report. Other surveys have shown that some interventional cardiologists make over $800,000 a year, with some neurosurgeons and cardiac surgeons earning over a million.[99]

In recent years, fewer medical students have chosen to become internists, pediatricians, or general practitioners (primary care), with lower compensation playing an important role. Lifestyle issues, such as hours of work and on-call schedules, are also factors. A report by the American Academy of Family Physicians in 2006 revealed that the number of medical school graduates who went into primary care medicine dropped by more than half from 1997 to 2005.[100] The report estimated that 39 percent more primary care physicians would be required in the United States by 2020. Another study proclaimed that nearly one in five Americans were "medically disenfranchised"—56 million people who lacked access to primary care physicians because of shortages in this field.[101] This deficiency was independent of insurance coverage. More than 1 million people in 21 different states had this problem, which was particularly acute in Florida, Texas, and California. An article in *U.S. News and World Report* in March 2008 noted that 29 percent of Medicare recipients had difficulty finding a doctor who would take their insurance (11.6 million people), two-thirds of Americans had trouble getting medical care on nights and weekends, and only 30 percent of Americans were able to get an appointment to see their physicians on the same day.[102] (Patients sometimes have to wait months to years for a routine physical.) Having health insurance doesn't mean much if you can't find a doctor when you're sick. (A shortage of general surgeons has also been reported recently in a study in the *Archives of Surgery*, causing problems at trauma centers, emergency departments, and rural hospitals.[103] This has occurred because more surgeons are choosing subspecialty fields where there are greater financial rewards.)

Ten years ago, half of all internal medicine residents went into primary care, whereas now just 20 percent do.[104] In addition to various subspecialties, many choose to become "hospitalists" who care for patients only during hospitalizations. Starting salaries for these physicians are around $200,000 or more, with no start-up practice costs, no problems with overhead, and fewer and better scheduled hours than those in private practice. Earnings are low for primary care physicians because Medicare and the insurance companies pay poorly for the kind of services they provide, which involves hands-on care, talking to patients, histories, and physicals, rather than well-compensated procedures. Because of the drop in U.S. students who opt for primary care, some of the slack has been picked up by foreign medical graduates. But the problem caused by a shortage of primary care physicians must be addressed if the quality of health care is to be improved.

Another issue to be considered is the level of students who are attracted to medicine in general, as well as to primary care. Medicine has traditionally appealed to many of the best and the brightest who excelled academically and were interested in research as well as clinical care. These were the individuals who were responsible for medical breakthroughs and became leaders in their fields. Today, more of the brightest college students are opting for careers in the financial field, or becoming entrepreneurs of one sort or another, rather than choosing medicine or science for their life's work.[105] The same loss of talent is true of academia, the law, and public service jobs, which are being bypassed by the young for the lure of material success and great wealth. (Perhaps this will change because of the current financial shake-up.) This is a societal issue transcending medicine that has no easy answers because it encompasses changing values. Interestingly, a recent report noted that residents in dermatology, plastic surgery, and otolaryngology (ENT) had the highest median medical board scores and the highest percentage of medical honor society membership among eighteen specialties.[106] These are fields involved in enhancing people's appearances, with the treatment of serious conditions a minor component. Again, the brightest students are abandoning the more challenging types of medical practice for a better lifestyle and higher compensation. (Many dermatologists have been found to extend preferential treatment to their cosmetic patients, who are much more lucrative to care for and usually pay in cash. They are often given earlier appointments, are seen in more luxurious settings, and are generally pampered.[107] These doctors would rather give Botox injections than diagnose and treat patients with melanoma and other potentially dangerous problems.)

As described in this chapter, there are a number of serious problems plaguing the health care system that are responsible for the evolving crisis. The escalating costs of care and the unfunded liabilities of the government are without doubt an immediate and long term threat to the U.S. economy. In addition, the large percentage of the population who are uninsured is a challenge to the nation's core beliefs in equality and justice. All of the flaws in the system contribute to its dysfunctionality, and all of them must be addressed together in a comprehensive reform plan.

## CHAPTER 5

# MALPRACTICE AND
# MEDICAL NEGLIGENCE

The need to compensate people for their injuries has long been recognized in most systems of law, and Western systems have a tradition of doing so by apportioning fault. The system's yin and yang of linking compensation of the injured to the fault of the injurer (hoping at the same time to deter future unsafe acts and do all of this fairly) is brilliant in its simplicity and works reasonably well when applied to many human endeavors.

Unfortunately, medicine is not one of them.[1]

The common law is at bottom the philosophy of pragmatism. Its truth is relative, not absolute.

—Justice Benjamin Cardozo[2]

In a conflict between two parties, an exemplary legal process would base a resolution on truth and justice; discovering the truth in the contested matter and finding a way to provide justice for both parties. However, the civil system in place in the United States that is charged with adjudicating malpractice cases is unconcerned with determining the truth and unable to deliver justice. Instead, both sides are primarily motivated by money. The plaintiff, and his or her attorneys, strive to maximize what they might gain, while the defendant and his or her advocates attempt to minimize what they might lose. These goals color the entire legal process, with truth and justice often its victim. "Studies undertaken in the 1980s and 1990s demonstrated convincingly that the current US system of medical malpractice litigation is expensive as a social policy and irrational as a compensatory mechanism."[3]

*Primum non nocerum.* Above all do no harm. This is the mantra physicians learn from the first day of medical school, which is repeated through their years of schooling and training. *Primum non nocerum.* No physician wants his or her actions, or lack of action, to result in injury to someone under his or her care. It is painful enough to have a patient who does poorly despite a doctor's ministrations and best efforts. But being responsible for injuring someone can be devastating to a physician emotionally and professionally.

Medical negligence indicates that an error has occurred in patient management because the usual standard of care was breached by that person's physician or other health care personnel. This may or may not result in harm to that individual. Malpractice and medical negligence are terms used almost synonymously, but negligence only becomes malpractice when trial lawyers enter the picture. Malpractice and medical negligence can be thought of as two sides of the same coin, bound together by the legal system. Unfortunately, medical negligence is a major problem confounding the delivery of health care, with far too many people being injured or dying because of medical errors. No one would argue against addressing this problem aggressively and reducing the incidence of negligence as much as possible. However, society must also be realistic. Medical care is provided by fallible human beings who may be distracted, tired, careless, or overburdened, and some mistakes are bound to occur.

Both medical negligence and malpractice independently drive up the costs of health care. Negligence also directly impacts individuals and families in terrifying ways, causing thousands of premature deaths and injuries annually, as patients are harmed by the caregivers to whom they turned for help. Since medical negligence can be so disastrous to its victims and their families, this problem should not be considered mainly in the context of its financial impact. Medical mistakes and negligence ruin people's lives and result in unnecessary suffering, and must be constrained for this reason alone. But heightened costs, of course, are also important. (In fact, there was an estimate 10 years ago that the total yearly costs related to medical errors could be as high as $200 billion.[4]) One of the ways medical negligence increases health care expenditures is through the treatment of iatrogenic (caused by physicians) illnesses or injuries, additional outlays that would not be required if the errors had not occurred. (Each adverse drug event in a hospital 10 years ago was calculated to result in $4,700 in additional expenditures.[5]) There is also the long term cost to society of caring for individuals who have been seriously injured while receiving treatment, and who may be disabled and no longer productive.

Various estimates have been made of the number of medical errors that occur each year, and the deaths and injuries that result. Most of the studies have been hospital-based—where the sickest patients are being treated, injuries are likely to be of greater severity, and the errors that cause them are easier to document. The Harvard Medical Practice Study in 1991 was a seminal report, analyzing hospitalized patients in New York state where negligence and adverse events were a consequence of care.[6] The authors found adverse events in 3.7 percent of hospitalizations, with 27.6 percent of these events felt to be the result of negligence. The percentage of these that caused permanent disabilities was 2.6, and 13.6

percent resulted in death. (Patients 65 or older were two to four times more likely to suffer medical injuries than those under age 45.) Extrapolating this study to all U.S. hospitals, one estimate had 120,000 Americans dying yearly from preventable errors in their hospital care.[7] However, there have been challenges to the accuracy of the Harvard Practice Study itself and the projections of medical negligence and deaths that followed, with some reports having much lower numbers. It appears that minor events in the study were weighted the same as more serious ones, and nonmedical occurrences (slip-and-falls) were counted with medical mistakes such as surgical errors.[8] In addition, many of the adverse events occurred in severely ill patients, some of whom were given high-risk treatments and who would have died within days anyway. To verify the results of the study, a second team of reviewers evaluated a small sample of the medical records. Although they found approximately the same number of adverse events and negligence as the first team, some of these were different events or in different patients, which raised some doubts about the data.[9] The Institute of Medicine in its important report *To Err Is Human*, in 1999 projected that 44,000 to 98,000 deaths occurred each year as a result of medical negligence.[10,11]

Though there may be questions about the actual number of incidents of medical negligence, as well as deaths and injuries that transpire in hospitals each year, there is little disagreement that the numbers are substantial. In 2000, the Institute of Medicine proposed a national undertaking to promote health care safety, recognizing that a major problem existed.[12] There was an emphasis on the need to modify the systems in place, as it was not just physicians whose missteps were responsible for negligence and adverse events. All hospital personnel were involved to varying degrees, including nurses, aides, technicians, pharmacists, and even transporters, with many of the problems that occurred being the result of poor communication. Physicians' orders may not have been completely legible or were interpreted the wrong way by a nurse. Or a pharmacist may have misread the dosage of a drug or added the wrong substance to an infusion. Or a technician might have injected contrast material for an imaging study into a patient who was allergic. Errors of this sort are evidence of systemic failings within the hospital and have to be corrected through quality control measures. (Some of these mistakes can be eliminated through the use of computerized charts and order sheets, with a patient's data being available to everyone in the hospital who is rendering care.) In 2007, Medicare published notices that it would no longer cover the extra costs of infections and other preventable adverse events in hospitalized patients.[13] It was hoped this policy would pressure hospitals to address these problems in a comprehensive fashion to save lives and reduce injuries, and that it would also lower Medicare expenditures. However, questions have been raised about whether Medicare will be able to select those complications which are truly preventable, as some of these problems may occur even with first-rate care.[14] The regulations may also lead physicians and hospitals to shy away from treating those patients who are sicker and more likely to develop complications while hospitalized.

Negligent actions also occur in physicians' offices and outpatient clinics, as well as other nonhospital health care facilities, through missteps by those personnel who have patient contact or who execute orders. Although some of these errors undoubtedly cause patient injuries and deaths, they are less likely to do so because most of the involved patients are less severely ill. The frequency of medical negligence and adverse events in outpatient settings is difficult to determine, given poor documentation, lack of accurate reporting, and attempts at concealment. A common claim in malpractice actions involving outpatient care is "failure to diagnose," where a physician overlooks a problem or reaches the wrong conclusion about a case that results in an injury to a patient.

When medical negligence is transformed into malpractice by plaintiffs' attorneys, health care costs are raised in different ways, while physicians suffer the prolonged emotional impact of the suits, regardless of whether they have done anything wrong. One way malpractice affects health care spending is through physicians' payments for professional liability coverage, the costs of which are passed on to patients (estimated to represent 15 percent of physicians services in 1987).[15] Since then, premiums for liability insurance have skyrocketed, without corresponding adjustments of the Resource Based Relative Value Scale (RBRVS) compensation schedule; the total cost of medical professional liability insurance in 2002 was calculated to be $25.6 billion.[16] The economic difficulties faced by many physicians because of the price of liability insurance cannot be overestimated. In some states, premiums have tripled since 2000 and may be in the hundreds of thousands for some specialists.[17] As examples, some internists in Cook County, Illinois paid over $50,000 for insurance in 2007, general surgeons over $127,000, and obstetricians over $178,000.[18] In Florida, the rates were even higher, with some general surgeons and obstetricians paying over $275,000. Though much of this is reflected in physicians' fees, there is just so much they are able to charge patients, particularly when Medicare and HMOs restrict their ability to raise fees. These exorbitant malpractice premiums have resulted in some physicians "going bare" (practicing without insurance) or closing their practices.

Defensive medicine, related to the fear of malpractice suits, is another factor that increases health care costs. When practicing defensive medicine, physicians order unnecessary tests to be certain that every unlikely cause for a problem is excluded. This is done to lessen the risk of a malpractice suit in the future, if they have made a wrong diagnosis. A CBS News report in 2007 mentioned that the cost of defensive medicine to the health care system is estimated to be more than $100 billion annually.[19] Another study calculated the costs in 2001 at between $69 billion and $124 billion.[20] Whatever the exact figure, it is evident that the number is significant and has contributed to ballooning health care costs. As an example of defensive medicine, when a patient comes into a hospital emergency room with a relatively minor head injury, the emergency physician invariably orders a CT scan of the head to be absolutely certain that no bleeding has occurred within the skull. This is not to help in diagnosis, but to protect the doctor from a malpractice action in the rare instance that a problem develops subsequently. An attorney can never question that doctor on the witness stand about why a CT scan was not obtained initially. (Not only does the test raise costs, but it also exposes the patient to unnecessary radiation.) The proper (cost-effective) way to manage this patient would be to follow him or her clinically and order a CT scan only if the signs or symptoms warranted it. But the emergency physician does not know what kind of follow-up the patient will have, so a CT scan is obtained, prematurely and unnecessarily. A survey of physicians several years ago showed that 79 percent ordered more tests than they deemed medically necessary in order to protect themselves from malpractice suits.[21]

Not only are excessive tests done for defensive reasons, but also invasive procedures and surgery. The above survey of physicians revealed that 51 percent recommended invasive procedures to confirm diagnoses more often than they believed were medically necessary.[22] Obviously, these can lead to complications and adverse events that can injure patients (and further raise costs). Inconsequential lesions may be biopsied to be sure they are not cancerous. Appendectomies may be performed on patients where the diagnosis is questionable to be certain the appendix will not rupture and cause peritonitis (an infection of the abdominal cavity), which may be more difficult to treat. Watchful waiting here might have produced an answer without surgery, but the surgeon didn't want to take the risk of being sued. Unnecessary Caesarian sections to deliver babies are also being done to protect obstetricians against malpractice suits associated with birth injuries. (Some of these operations are also done for convenience or to boost fees.) Personal injury attorneys have focused on birth injuries with lifelong consequences as the types of cases that can generate huge awards because of sympathetic juries, regardless of whether the physicians' actions met or did not meet the standard of care.

Another manifestation of defensive medicine is increased referrals to specialists. The same survey that was previously cited also noted that 74 percent of physicians referred to specialists more often than they considered medically necessary to try and protect themselves.[23]

Physicians are also more likely to see patients in their offices or emergency rooms for minor problems that could be handled with phone calls, just to be sure that nothing is missed. In addition, patients with questionable symptoms are sent to emergency rooms to be evaluated by emergency physicians if their regular doctor is unable to see them. There is an unwillingness by doctors to risk a bad outcome in any patient, even if the likelihood is extremely remote. This type of mind-set does not consider cost effectiveness.

Partially, because of defensive medicine, physicians have gotten into the habit of ordering unnecessary tests, doing unnecessary procedures, and referring out to specialists even when malpractice actions are not a consideration. These ingrained habits may be hard to break if and when malpractice reform ever makes defensive medicine moot. Doctors may have to be educated to a new way of thinking.

Aside from the issue of increased costs, malpractice suits negatively impact medical care in other ways.

1. Physicians are reluctant to take on complex cases. Aside from referrals to specialists, if there is a greater likelihood of a bad outcome, primary care physicians or surgeons may shunt off patients to other PCPs or surgeons and simply not start with these individuals because of their concern about the possibility of malpractice suits. In some areas, obstetricians are reluctant to deliver babies and only do gynecology because of the high cost of obstetrical malpractice insurance and the risk of large malpractice awards when there are problems with pregnancies or deliveries.

2. Fewer physicians will be available in the coming years in states with high premiums for malpractice insurance and those that have the most suits. New physicians do not want to open practices in these states, even as older ones are leaving or retiring. This means that patients in these areas will have less access to medical care, particularly in high risk specialties such as obstetrics, neurosurgery, and orthopedics.

3. Medical students will be choosing specialties where they are less likely to be sued. Consequently, patients may be unable to obtain care in vital fields in the future.

4. Physicians are hesitant to see Medicaid or indigent patients, or work in clinics. They don't want exposure to additional patients (who may sue them) with little or no compensation for their efforts. (However, some studies have shown that poor and uninsured patients are less likely to sue for malpractice after medical injuries than the population at large.[24])

5. Fewer good students will pick medicine as a career, knowing that their income will be reduced because of the cost of malpractice insurance, and they will have an increased likelihood of being sued and winding up in court.

6. Physician-patient relationships will be increasingly poisoned by the specter of malpractice that hangs over any dealings they may have. Some physicians see patients as potential sources of litigation and are wary in their dealings with them.

7. Physicians have a higher anxiety level when managing patients and work under more stress, making it more difficult for them to perform well.

It is evident that medical negligence and malpractice increase health care costs and reduce access to care for many patients. The questions that must be asked are: what is the best way to attack medical negligence and malpractice? Is the current system effective and only in need of some small adjustments to improve it? Is the current approach so flawed that it needs to be completely overhauled?

Any program designed to address medical negligence and malpractice (either alone or as a part of comprehensive health care reform) should have five main objectives:

1. Decreasing the incidence of medical negligence.
2. Properly and rationally compensating individuals who have been significantly injured as a result of negligence.

3. Removing incompetent physicians from patient care.
4. Punishing physicians who are repeatedly guilty of negligence.
5. Instituting a process both patients and physicians believe is equitable and swift.

The current methods of handling malpractice and negligence through legal redress have failed to meet any of the above objectives. The system now in place, using lawsuits to compensate patients for injuries due to medical negligence, is both ineffective and wasteful. A report in the *New England Journal of Medicine* on assessing patients who had sued for malpractice, found upon review that there was no correlation between adverse events caused by negligence and payment to patients.[25] Interestingly, 10 of 24 cases, where the reviewers had determined no adverse events due to negligence had occurred, were settled in favor of the plaintiffs, as well as 6 of 13 cases where there had been adverse events but no negligence (which is called maloccurrence: a bad outcome where no one is at fault). This is merely one report of how poorly the malpractice system works and why lawyers are willing to pursue some actions that seem tenuous at best. Another study noted that only 1.53 percent of patients injured by medical negligence ever filed a claim, and only 8–13 percent of these cases went to trial.[26] In addition, only 1.2–1.9 percent were decided for the plaintiffs.[27] Yet, almost $25,000 was spent, on average, by the insurance companies and defendants to defend each claim, no matter how frivolous or minor it may have been.[28] The process of malpractice suits to compensate injured patients is long, laborious, inefficient, expensive, and too frequently results in inappropriate outcomes.

The present system also does not address the general issue of negligence or improving the quality of care. When malpractice lawyers win or lose a particular case, it does not transform the practice of medicine in any way or even impact the particular facet of care that was legally contested. And many cases where malpractice was clear cut are settled without the defendant physician having to admit negligence. Attorneys claim that the fear of malpractice suits keeps physicians on their toes and makes them less likely to be negligent. But there is no evidence this is so (though the threat does increase health care costs by encouraging defensive medicine.) Even those physicians found in court to have committed malpractice are still able to practice without oversight. Only repeated suits may cause a physician to be watched by the state authorities or to possibly have his or her license suspended. As the lawyer Winston Hubert Smith noted in writing about medical malpractice, "The civil action for damages enforces only incidentally the standards of medical practice."[29]

(In 1986, Congress established the National Practitioner Data Bank [NPDB] as part of the Health Care Quality Improvement Act. This was to be an electronic record of all malpractice awards or settlements made against physicians or other health care practitioners, as well as negative actions stemming from peer review, loss or suspension of licenses, hospital privileges, or professional society memberships.[30] This information was to be available upon request to state licensing boards, professional societies, hospitals, and other health care entities. To date, the NPDB does not appear to have affected the incidence of medical negligence or malpractice, nor improved the quality of care. The data has come mainly from malpractice awards, which does not correlate with physician competence.)

Though there are numerous instances of suboptimal care by physicians and other caregivers that must be dealt with, medical negligence often results from systemic problems that have to be addressed systemically to reduce the frequency of errors. Changes have to occur in the process by which patients receive care, with insightful analysis to discover the areas where mistakes are made and then to correct them. And physicians who are prone to errors have to be scrutinized more carefully, have further education, supervision if necessary, with the ultimate loss of their medical licenses if it is felt they remain at risk.

Malpractice actions in the current system do not decrease the incidence of medical negligence, they do not adequately compensate injured patients, they do not remove incompetent physicians, and they usually do not punish those guilty of negligence. The suits are simply a lottery system devised by attorneys, where a small number of injured patients benefit. Advertising by trial lawyers, who want to attract personal injury cases, persuades individuals who are angry at physicians or hospitals or dissatisfied with the outcome of their care, to use the lawyer's services. The attorneys make it seem as if their prime interest is their client's welfare, reinforced by statements that they will charge no fee for taking a case, and that their payment will come from any damages recovered. Ads may be found in newspapers, on the radio, and television, with displays often prominent in subways, buses, and on billboards, enticing people with the possibility of found money if they pursue an action. Those who feel they have been injured or wronged may see a big payout ahead, and those with minor injuries are encouraged to magnify them to increase any awards that might be obtained. A study in the Annals of Internal Medicine in 1994 showed that the most frequent reason for initiating a suit given by callers who contacted attorney's offices about possible malpractice actions was television advertising, noted by 73 percent.[31] (Twenty-five percent of these individuals had previously been involved in other litigation, excluding divorce.)

Specialists, who often deal with the more difficult cases where there may be poor outcomes, are more likely to be sued by patients or their families than are primary care physicians. But it is not just the outcomes that drive malpractice suits. As patients and families do not have lengthy relationships with most specialists, they are more prone to bring actions against them if they are unhappy with the results of their care. On the other hand, primary care physicians with long-standing connections to their patients and families are less likely to be sued, even when they have made mistakes. In general, doctors who are warm, outgoing, and interact well with their patients, rarely wind up in court. Communication and relationships with the patients and families may be as important, or more so, than whether or not negligence has occurred. One review of malpractice cases revealed that patients most often decided to sue when they perceived a lack of caring and concern on the part of the doctor when there were adverse events.[32] Of course, the way patients and their families view their physician in terms of compassion and understanding may also color their opinion about his or her competence.

Recently, there has been a sea change in the way physicians have been advised to react when medical mistakes occur. Previously, physicians and hospitals went to unusual lengths to try and conceal any errors, particularly if they resulted in injuries, afraid that their admissions would result in malpractice suits. Now, it is recommended by many quality-of-care organizations that physicians disclose errors to patients and families, take responsibility for them, and apologize.[33] It is believed that malpractice suits will be less likely if this path is followed, where patient anger may be assuaged by physicians who are sympathetic figures and are willing to communicate. There have also been some legislative proposals regarding disclosure linked with early compensation for patients who have been injured, but nothing has yet been enacted.

The problem of the escalating cost of malpractice insurance to physicians and its potential effect on access to care, with special attention to so-called high-risk specialties such as obstetrics and neurosurgery, has been in the news for a number of years. During this period, Congress has been unable to craft any solutions, and there has been little legislative relief on a state level. However, physician unhappiness with the malpractice system was simmering for decades, even before insurance rates began to soar. Physicians were angered by what they perceived as a lack of equity in the malpractice process and the belief that they could not obtain justice when an action was brought against them, thus losing from a financial and emotional standpoint even if a jury or court decided in their favor.

If a physician defendant is found guilty of malpractice by a jury, or settles the case because the weight of evidence is against him or her, he or she is a big loser. (Insurance companies in some instances are able to force physicians to settle cases if the company thinks it will be less expensive than mounting a defense.) Physicians may also decide to settle even if they believe there was no malpractice, out of fear that a jury may award the plaintiff more than their insurance coverage, making them personally liable. In each of these situations, the physician is a big loser, with malpractice insurance more difficult to obtain, or premiums being raised.

On the other hand, if the jury finds in favor of the physician defendant after a trial, or the case is dismissed by the judge or withdrawn by the plaintiff's attorney before coming to trial, then the physician is only a small loser and is supposed to walk away happy. He or she has gone through years of stress (cases often linger 7–10 years before reaching trial), has been accused of all sorts of nefarious activities, and has lost weeks or months of productive time reviewing medical records, giving testimony in depositions, and possibly attending a trial. Yet, there is no way for the physician to obtain compensation for the time and money he or she has lost, much less for the distress suffered. And the medical liability insurance companies may have spent thousands to hundreds of thousands of dollars to mount a defense for the accused physician, necessitating further increases in all physicians' premiums. Even in egregiously unfair or frivolous cases, physicians are unable to countersue the plaintiff or his or her attorney for damages sustained, unless they are willing to pay up front, as no attorney will take these cases on a contingency basis. Unlike plaintiffs who bring malpractice actions and don't have to advance any money to their lawyers, physicians have to pay attorneys an hourly rate if they wish to sue to recover damages.

It is possible for a physician defendant to lose his or her home and life savings—everything he or she has worked for—in a malpractice suit. This scenario may be increasingly common in the future as the amount of coverage offered by medical liability companies drops in response to rising awards by juries and heightened costs, in spite of spiraling premiums. The juries that hand down these awards and the general population are usually not aware of this possibility, which is, of course, extremely frightening to physicians. At times, this fear leads to settlements within the limits of their coverage, even though they believe they have done nothing wrong.

Aside from the issue of equity, frustrated physicians view the entire malpractice process as flawed, knowing that only chance (and not good medical practice) keeps them from its clutches. They understand that malpractice suits are not about the problem of medical negligence and are not an attempt to bring about necessary changes. Instead, these actions are opportunities for plaintiffs and trial lawyers to obtain large payouts in cases where the treatment was unsuccessful or the results failed to meet expectations, whether or not there was actual malpractice. All that a plaintiff's attorney needs to bring an action is to find another doctor with similar training to the defendant who will say that the standard of care was breached, which is merely that person's opinion. Physician defendants, who are perceived as affluent, and their insurance companies are seen as vulnerable adversaries with deep pockets by attorneys—adversaries who usually do not evince compassion from jurors. And plaintiffs' counsels will do whatever they can to denigrate and disparage physician defendants in front of the jurors.

In addition, malpractice cases require complex medical testimony to be given before a lay jury whose members often do not comprehend the issues before them. The jurors usually have to listen to dueling expert witnesses from both the plaintiffs and defendants, then try to decide what has transpired. The skill of the attorneys and the experts on both sides may determine how the jury votes, rather than the true merits of the case. And experts can always be found to bolster an attorney's arguments, if he or she is willing to pay for them. In fact, there is an industry of expert witnesses who charge $500 to $1,000 an hour and are willing to testify on any aspect of a case. Unfortunately, the jury is often unable to decipher the testimony of the opposing experts who present contradictory viewpoints, biased in favor of their patrons, with no attempt at impartiality or seeking the truth. The noted trial lawyer Melvin Belli once said, "If I got myself an impartial witness, I'd think I was wasting my money."[34]

Cases are frequently decided on emotional grounds, with the plaintiff's attorney using a bad outcome as evidence of malpractice, perhaps parading a paralyzed or damaged patient in the courtroom to win the jury's sympathy without proving that the standard of care was breached. (We have shown previously that experts have determined in post hoc reviews that no malpractice is committed in many cases that are decided for the plaintiffs.) Adding to physicians' perceptions of unfairness is the fact that the judges who control the process may have been trial lawyers before being appointed to the bench, and their rulings frequently reflect their backgrounds. The entire process is tilted in favor of the plaintiff.

Successful ventures encourage other similar ventures in the United States. Thus, success in malpractice actions begets new ones. Patients or their families see or hear that someone has made millions of dollars with a suit for a medical injury. They are unhappy with the outcome of their treatment for a particular affliction and possibly with their relationship with their physician. So they find lawyers willing to take their case, which gives them an opportunity to make some money or get back at their physician. At times, the fact that a poor outcome is to be expected as part of the natural history of the illness may be ignored.

Lawyers accept some cases hoping to achieve quick settlements with the insurance carrier, knowing that defending a suit in court will be much more costly to that company. With a minimum of effort, they may be able to obtain tens of thousands of dollars. And if it does come to court, a sympathetic jury may give them a verdict even if no negligence has occurred. There is also no consistency to the amount of awards in malpractice cases and no logic or standards to make it predictable. It depends on the persuasiveness of the attorneys, the emotions and whims of the jury, sympathy for the plaintiff, and anger against the physician. Large awards without legally proscribed limits are increasingly common and further distort the system, especially when given for noneconomic damages (pain and suffering, loss of consortium, loss of enjoyment of life, etc.).

Part of the problem is also that there is a patchwork of malpractice laws from state to state, with some offering a cap on noneconomic damages, some having panels of experts that review cases, and others with various, individualized nonstandard statutes. Noneconomic damages make up a major portion of the awards in some states. Thus, some states may be low cost in terms of malpractice insurance, while others are astronomically high, completely contingent upon their laws. This lack of uniformity makes it difficult for insurance companies to assess risk and write polices and drives up administrative expenses. In today's malpractice climate, it also means that more and more physicians will be gravitating towards those states whose laws they see as being physician-friendly.

As the attorney Philip Howard noted in his book *The Death of Common Sense*, "Modern law is a game of parsing and logical intrigue. Whenever detailed provisions bend and twist, the observant lawyer will find a place where he can go and violate the spirit of the rules, or get an advantage over others, and do so with complete impunity."[35] Trial lawyers are the force propping up the current malpractice system and the ones who derive the most benefit from it. Because their income is tied directly to the process that adjudicates malpractice claims, they have been fighting tooth and nail to maintain the present way that claims are handled. But because a system has been functioning for many years does not mean it is the best way to accomplish an objective or that it should be continued indefinitely. Contrary to the overwhelming evidence that favors change, trial lawyers have been obstructing all attempts at malpractice reform, using every avenue open to them. This includes contributing large sums to the campaign funds of politicians, expressly directing their largess to key legislators on both state and national levels.

The Trial Lawyers Association also has lobbyists actively working with Congress and state legislatures to prevent any critical statutes affecting malpractice from being passed. (The Association of Trial Lawyers changed its name to the American Association for Justice after a number of its most prominent members went to jail for subverting the legal process in various ways.) Walter K. Olson, an authority on tort reform, noted in 2003 that "For twenty years, there has been talk of action in Washington to reform the excesses of the liability system and rein in the power of trial lawyers. And over twenty years, little if any reform of any real significance has made it to enactment at the federal level. . . . The litigation lobby rightly boasts of its record, year in and year out, under Republicans and Democrats alike, of turning back any threats to its prosperity."[36] Reinforcing lobbying efforts by personal injury lawyers against malpractice reform, large numbers of legislators also happen to be lawyers in the forefront of the battle to maintain the status quo.

In addition, the Trial Lawyers Association places advertisements on television, radio, and the print media designed to sway public opinion against malpractice reform. They use examples of egregious medical negligence resulting in injuries or deaths to win sympathy for their cause, omitting statistics about how few victims of negligence are actually compensated under the current system, and how valuable it is to the pocketbooks of trial attorneys.

Adding to physicians' frustration over the system in place is their inability to discipline their own: to cull out those bad apples who are repeatedly negligent because of ignorance, carelessness, or illness. While these bad apples are only part of the problem of medical negligence, and systemic breakdowns may be more important, attorneys and the legal system have made it nearly impossible under the peer review process for doctors to address those responsible for recurring medical errors in an effective fashion. Common sense would dictate that physicians themselves would be the ones to control incompetent physicians, and there is a moral obligation to do so as well. But there are no "safe harbors" for doctors who are whistle-blowers or those who sit on peer review bodies. There is always a threat of legal action by the physician being scrutinized, claiming slander or noncompetitive practices. Since that threat hangs over any disciplinary action, useful measures are blocked, given that no physician wants to suffer through the rigors of defending him or herself against a suit, even when the facts are clear-cut and the likelihood of winning is high.

Consumer groups and trial lawyers frequently complain that physicians are unwilling to testify against other physicians in depositions or at trials, even when those practitioners may be medically negligent. They say that doctors try to stonewall to protect their colleagues in all situations. Though this is true to some degree, it is because physicians view the malpractice process as blatantly unfair and don't want to be involved with it in any way. They want to rid the profession of incompetent practitioners, but feel physicians should be judged by their peers who understand what is involved with medical decision-making and not by lay juries who may be swayed by eloquent attorneys and emotional arguments.

There is an old story of a lawyer who comes to a town and puts out a shingle anticipating a flood of clients as there are no other lawyers around. But business is slow for some time until a second lawyer settles in the area. Within a short period, business is booming for both of them. This is the way the legal system works: attorneys generate business for other attorneys for which the general population pays.

The current method of handling presumed malpractice by physicians and other health care providers is a waste of time and resources, in addition to being completely ineffective. It is unfair to both physicians and patients. There are far better ways to deal with the issue of medical negligence, from the standpoints of trying to correct the problem of negligence, improve health care quality, and compensating victims who have been injured. Present attempts at reform at both the state and federal levels have focused on capping awards for noneconomic damages and have not addressed the lack of equity, which is like trying to put bandages on a festering wound instead of debriding it and cutting away the infected tissue. Transforming the malpractice system now in place must be an integral part of comprehensive health care reform.

## CHAPTER 6

# COMPREHENSIVE HEALTH CARE REFORM

> Observe constantly that all things come about by change; accustom yourself to reflect that the nature of the universe loves nothing so much as changing things that are and making new things like them. For everything that exists is in a way the seed of what will be.

> —Marcus Aurelius, *Meditations*[1]

Health care reform needs to address two problems at the heart of the current crisis: runaway costs that threaten to subvert the economy and the number of Americans without health insurance. As previously mentioned, the economic consequences will be devastating if health care costs are not contained. Projections have U.S. spending on health care reaching $4 trillion annually in 2016 and comprising 20 percent of GDP.[2] Estimates of the government's unfunded liabilities linked to Medicare and Medicaid range up to tens of trillions of dollars. The hospital trust fund, Medicare Part A, faces bankruptcy by 2019, or even earlier, if there are no corrective measures to prevent it.[3] In fact, if spending on health care maintains the same trajectory it is now following, the point will be reached some time in the next several decades where the annual increase in the U.S. GDP will go entirely for health care.[4] And alarmingly, the economist Laurence Kotlikoff believes the projections for the unfunded liabilities of Medicare and Medicaid and the growth rate for health care spending may be too conservative.[5]

In advanced societies, when people are unable to obtain medical coverage, there are consequences both for those individuals and the society, with increased morbidity and mortality and diminished productivity. As important as the economic aspects of the health care crisis are, providing universal access to care should be regarded as a moral issue, with the endorsement of health care as a basic human right. The United States is the only developed country that does not guarantee all of its citizens affordable care, and it is time this glaring omission was corrected. Comprehensive health care reform will not only help those individuals now lacking medical coverage, but will raise the quality of care for everyone, and be a boon to businesses and society. But it will not be easy. A recent article in the *Journal of the American Medical Association* noted that "At the heart of the challenge is transforming a nineteenth century craft-oriented delivery system to provide 21st century biomedical science and technology."[6]

However, there is also a concern by many citizens about the cost of reforming health care in these financially turbulent times, regarding how it might be funded. To allay this concern, there is convincing evidence (which will be presented shortly) that comprehensive reform with universal access to care can be achieved without *any* increase in the current spending for health care. No additional funding would be necessary. In fact, if properly constituted, reform can save the United States and its citizens considerable amounts of money, while delivering quality care. Unfortunately, it will require a knockdown, drag-out battle with the special interests who don't want comprehensive reform and have much to lose in money and power if the program is enacted. But with both the United States' economic and personal health on the line, reform is a necessity. Enacting the crucial changes will also entail battling the free-market ideologues in Congress and the media who see the market as the proper vehicle for reform. But it *must* be done.

As has been noted, there are three major elements required for any program of health care reform to be successful. These are simplification, universal (or near universal) access to care, and realistic cost constraints. A fourth element may also be added: severing the connection between health care coverage and employment, which is bad for businesses and tethers individuals to their jobs. Given that these criteria are necessary for a workable program, the current health care system must be thoroughly overhauled, since it does not meet any of them. In fact, it has failed dramatically in every area.

And once a new system has been established, a way must also be found to restrict political influence from the operative decisions relating to health care, which have thus far been both costly and destructive. Over the years, lobbyists and special interests have been able to weave their seductive spell over Congress and various federal agencies to shape the laws and regulations to meet their own needs rather than those of patients and society. Accelerated spending on health care will never be controlled while politics remains in the driver's seat.

The fear of U.S. citizens regarding significant changes to the health care system must also be assuaged if an effective program is to be enacted. Those who are satisfied with their health insurance must be made to understand that a major transformation of the system is mandatory or its cost will eventually overwhelm them, their children, and succeeding generations. They must also be assured that their relationships with favored physicians will not be torn asunder by any new program, and that the quality of care will only improve over time, given better oversight and the elimination of unnecessary care. Their fear of government involvement in health care, which has been labeled "socialized medicine" by opponents of change, must also be allayed. This will come with the appreciation that Medicare under government aegis has been a great success story for those individuals 65 and older, and that even now the government funds nearly two-thirds of the nation's total health care spending. Socialized medicine is merely a name placed on the process by the enemies of reform. And comprehensive reform is not predicated on government control of health care.

(A survey of physicians in March and April 2008 found that 95 percent of them favored reform of the health care system.[7] Three possible structures for reform were cited almost equally: a universal health insurance system with a single payer, a universal system with multiple payers, and tax credits for the uninsured to purchase coverage.)

In formulating a program of health care reform, there are a number of issues that need to be addressed: Who is to be covered by the program? How will it be funded? Who will administer the program, collect and disburse the funds, and provide oversight? How will cost constraints be effected? Who will decide which services will be covered? What role should the market play? What role should the government play? Should profit-oriented insurance companies continue to control the system. If not, what should their role be?

## Components of Comprehensive Health Care Reform

The essential elements of a comprehensive program for health care reform are outlined below. The reasons for each, how they would be accomplished, and how they would all be integrated will be subsequently described in more detail, along with some of the lesser components of the program.

1. Extension of Medicare to include all Americans and provide universal access to health care. This "Universal Medicare" would be transformed into an *independent* government-sponsored entity that is free from political interference.
2. Universal Medicare (UM) would be constituted as a single-payer system.
3. Universal Medicare would be under the control of a Federal Medicare Board (FMB, similar to the Federal Reserve Board), its members nominated by the president and approved by the Senate, and serving lengthy, staggered terms. The FMB would be assisted in its operations by at least seven standing advisory committees of experts in various fields, including therapeutics, diagnostics, preventive medicine, hospitals, oversight, administration and organizational matters, and provider reimbursement and salaries. There would also be District Medical Boards to assist the FMB.
4. The funding of Universal Medicare would come from multiple sources: enrollee premiums, the current Medicare tax, business contributions, deductibles and co-pays, and state and federal government contributions. Medigap insurance would provide additional coverage (Tier 2). For those who wanted every medical option for care, or to be treated by nonparticipating private physicians, Tier 3 insurance would be available.

5. Universal Medicare would have a fixed budget as a set percentage of the nation's GDP and would have to live within those limits.

6. Physicians would be salaried to eliminate incentives for unnecessary tests and procedures, as well as billing fraud. The differential in income between primary care physicians and procedure-oriented specialists would be reduced. Hospital reimbursement would continue to be based on a prospective payment system related to discharge diagnosis.

7. Medical education and training would be subsidized.

8. There would be regional health entities (RHEs) managing care for population bases of 1–5 million people in different geographic areas. They would employ physicians and other health care providers and would be responsible for delivering care to patients. These entities would have service contracts from Universal Medicare and would not profit from providing or withholding care.

9. Electronic health records (EHRs) would be established for all patients, with every physician and health care provider having computer terminals with compatible, interoperable software to access the data in their offices.

10. Physician extenders (nurse practitioners and physicians' assistants) would be utilized to help provide services, particularly in the area of preventive care.

11. Malpractice reform would be instituted to eliminate defensive medicine and provide quick and fair compensation to injured patients in appropriate circumstances.

## Extension of Medicare

The United States already has a program in place that provides health care coverage for about one-seventh of the population, with its reach projected to extend to one-fifth over the next several decades. It is called Medicare, with close to universal access to health care for older people (and the covered disabled) under the program. The infrastructure for this program already exists and is working well. Extending Medicare to the entire population of the United States (with some important modifications to insure that costs will be held in check and removing it from direct government control) would appear to be the easiest and most direct path to universal care. (Medicare also happens to be a single-payer system for the population it covers. An article in 2003 by Jonathan Oberlander noted that Medicare, "shares the main properties of the single-payer model: universality for its population, government-operated insurance, and centralized control."[8])

There will be strenuous objections by all the health care industry players to this approach, since it seems to be based on greater government involvement (or at least a centralized structure). However, providing coverage to all Americans instead of just some Americans by the government, or a government-backed entity, is only a matter of degree. It is illogical for opponents of national health insurance to accept current Medicare as a reasonable option for part of the population, yet reject its extension to the entire population (except on the basis of self-interest). Other government health care programs such as Medicaid, Federal

Employees Health Benefits Program (FEHBP), State Children's Health Insurance Program (SCHIP), VA benefits, and Indian health care would all be absorbed into this new entity which would be called Universal Medicare (UM). This strategy, if followed, would help to simplify the entire process of health care coverage, though, of course, the devil is in the details of how this would be done.

It must be kept in mind that in every country in the Organization for Economic Cooperation and Development (OECD), other than the United States, the government completely controls health care expenditures, from hiring and paying the physicians and other providers, funding the hospitals, buying equipment and pharmaceuticals, and so on.[9] In regard to the present health care system in the United States, which supposedly is dominated by the free market, an article in the *New England Journal of Medicine* in 1999 noted that "Government spending for health care in the United States—. . . including insurance premiums for government employees and tax subsidies for private insurance—exceeds total per capita health care spending in every other nation except Switzerland."[10] In other words, the government already is the major source of funding for U.S. health care in a fragmented, inefficient private system that must be drastically changed.

Though the opportunity to enroll in Universal Medicare would be extended to all Americans, participation would not be mandated initially, as envisioned by some of the health plans being circulated. Rather than forcing Americans to purchase coverage, the key to the Universal Medicare plan would be in making it attractive enough in terms of cost, convenience, and benefits to entice almost everyone to sign up voluntarily. Nevertheless, there are some who would not enroll, which is why it should be thought of as providing near universal access to care. But the ability to obtain coverage and care would be available to every American. (It is of course possible that if enough people did not sign up for Universal Medicare, notwithstanding its attractiveness, the program would at some point have to be made mandatory.)

All citizens and legal residents of the country could enroll in this program which would provide basic health care coverage similar to current Medicare benefits for older Americans. (Medicare Part A now covers hospitalization; Part B medical benefits: physicians charges, physical therapy, occupational therapy, etc.; Part C is Medicare Advantage: HMOs; and Part D is drug benefits. These programs would be integrated into UM.) There would be no more cherry-picking of enrollees by insurance companies or experiential rating. There would be no more denials of coverage because of preexisting conditions. There would be no more obstacles to medically indicated care. There would be new found freedom for employees to maximize career possibilities and move from job to job if they so desired, without worrying about health insurance and portability. People could retire prior to age 65 unconcerned about COBRA and maintaining health care coverage. Genetic testing would no longer be precluded by possible rejections for insurance, as people would no longer be penalized for hereditary predispositions to illness. In fact, obtaining health insurance would be fairly automatic for anyone who wanted it and no longer a source of anxiety. With this new method of coverage, U.S. businesses would not be burdened by health insurance costs that reduce their competitiveness in the global economy. There would be no more negotiations with insurance companies about providing coverage or worries about self-insurance. And health benefits would not be an issue that corporations would contest with their unions.

In addition to providing universal or near universal access to care, extending Medicare benefits to all Americans would best meet the reform objective of simplicity and efficiency compared to other proposals that are being advanced. Universal Medicare would protect all Americans with the same basic coverage and would not require them to have to decipher different plans. However, as is true with current Medicare, private insurance companies could offer supplemental coverage (Medigap coverage) over and beyond the basic plan, paying for the costs of *covered* services that UM did not. Medigap would handle out-of-pocket costs such as co-pays and deductibles, as well as providing extra benefits to those who enrolled. Different plans might furnish additional days of hospitalization, more extensive physical therapy, more covered days of rehabilitation, skilled nursing home benefits, foreign travel emergency care, and so forth, than would be available under the basic plan. However, the number of supplemental plans allowed to be marketed by the insurance companies would be limited (perhaps 12 as is now the case: Plans A to L), with benefit packages the same in comparable plans proffered by different companies. In other words, the plans would be standardized, with Plan A offered by various insurance companies all the same. Plan B would all be exactly the same across the board. This is the way Medigap is presently set up, permitting enrollees to compare apples to apples instead of having to deal with a confusing array of plans with a plethora of benefits. Insurance companies would have to compete for customers with the same plans (as is now being done with Medigap policies) on the basis of price and convenience.

Medigap plans would first be sold to individuals by insurance companies at the time Universal Medicare became effective, with no denials for preexisting conditions if they signed up at the initial offering. The insurance companies would not be permitted to drop a person's coverage for any reason other than nonpayment of premiums. Enrollees would be allowed to switch Medigap companies to try and get lower costs or more benefits only during the open enrollment periods, which would be established for one month each year. (Consideration might have to be given to making government subsidies available to assist lower income people in purchasing Medigap policies.)

These supplemental insurance plans would also not be mandatory and not everyone would obtain them. With basic coverage guaranteed by Universal Medicare, some people might elect to take a chance that they would not need the extra benefits and therefore not purchase Medigap, hoping to save money if they were not sick. However, if they did not join at the beginning, they could only opt in subsequently during open enrollment periods and might have to pay the higher premiums or face a waiting period. These Medigap supplemental insurance plans would be known as Universal Medicare, Tier 2.

(Another consideration would be to eliminate Medigap completely and have Universal Medicare pay all the costs and charges of health care. This would require higher premiums for enrollees and increases from other sources of funding. Though this action would further simplify the system, the rise in basic costs, the avoidance of any individual responsibility, and the lack of freedom for enrollees to choose other coverages makes it less enticing.)

In addition to the Medigap plans, insurance companies would be permitted to market a level of coverage known as Tier 3. These plans would provide benefits over and above what Universal Medicare covered. They would be aimed at those individuals who wanted every possible treatment and diagnostic option open to them no matter what their age or condition might be, whether or not the treatment was considered effective by a UM evaluation board, and independent of any cost/benefit ratio. (The services that will be covered by Universal Medicare will be discussed subsequently.) Tier 3 coverage would not be regulated by UM, and the insurance companies would not be obligated to present standardized plans at competitive costs. The companies could structure the plans any way they wanted and price them however they saw fit. A multitude of different plans could be offered to the public with different benefits, co-pays, deductibles, and so forth. Though these plans would provide more inclusive services than Universal Medicare, the added measures would not necessarily result in better care for those who signed up. (Appropriate care, determined by UM's Committee on Therapeutics, would already be covered.) Tier 3 plans would undoubtedly be expensive and likely to be purchased only by affluent individuals.

Tier 3 plans might also offer enrollees coverage for private care by physicians who were not participants in Universal Medicare and who wanted to practice outside of a government-supported program. (Freedom of choice to join or reject UM would have to be offered to physicians, as well as consumers of health care.) These private physicians could accept Tier 3 insurance for their services or insist on direct payment, with the insurance companies reimbursing patients for their out-of-pocket costs. This type of care would be similar to what is currently known as "boutique medicine." (Participants in Tier 3 coverage would still have to pay their UM premiums.)

## Single-Payer System

As simplicity and reduced administrative costs must be part of any reform program, a single-payer system is mandatory. A single-payer system has been proposed in the past as the primary component of health care reform,[11,12] but without adequate control of costs on the provider's side of the equation. There are estimates that changing to a single-payer system could save as much as $350 billion annually that is now spent on the medical bureaucracy.[13] However, some economists believe that this change would merely shift the overhead costs rather than reduce them.[14] They argue that monitoring of services, which is now performed by the administrative staff of the private insurance companies, would have to be assumed by the single-payer to control excessive care. But if physician incentives to provide unnecessary services were eliminated as a part of comprehensive reform (which will be discussed subsequently), then careful monitoring would no longer be required.

The single-payer should not be the government itself, or one of its branches, but an autonomous government-backed entity, that is, Universal Medicare, separate from the Department of Health and Human Services. Having it function independently is a necessity. Establishing Universal Medicare in this fashion would help shield it from the political pressure and interference that have played a major role in the escalation of health care costs. Universal Medicare would be vested with responsibility by Congress for all aspects of health care in the United States, but would not be directly under its supervision. (Universal Medicare might be considered as a hybrid of the Federal Reserve Board and a government-sponsored enterprise similar to the Federal Home Loan Mortgage Association (Fannie Mae). Though Fannie Mae recently imploded and was taken over by the government because of imprudent management and lack of oversight, it performed effectively for many years to help U.S. home ownership grow. It got into trouble when its lobbyists pressured Congress to allow it to act in a risky manner, and when it tried to enhance its profits and compensation to its top executives. To forestall any abuses, the executives of Universal Medicare would be paid a fixed salary, perhaps allowing bonuses pegged to cost savings and quality improvement. There would be no incentives tied to profit, as that was responsible for the fraud, "cooking of the books," and foolish risk-taking at Fannie Mae and Freddie Mac. There would also be strict oversight at every level.)

## Federal Medicare Board

Universal Medicare would be run by a board similar to the Federal Reserve Board, its members appointed by the president and confirmed by the Senate. It would have 11 members, 9 of them regular appointees, in addition to a chairman and vice-chairman. To mitigate against political interference with its actions, members would be appointed for lengthy terms (8 or 10 years), and to ensure continuity of its functions, the terms would be staggered, with two or three board members appointed every two years. (If a member died in office, was incapacitated, or resigned for any reason, the new appointment would merely fill the remainder of his or her term.) It is hoped that appointees chosen by the president would be nonpartisan technocrats, selected for their expertise rather than their political leanings, and would include administrators, physicians, economists, and business people. Like the "Fed," the Federal Medicare Board (FMB) would be a powerful entity, being charged with running 16–20 percent of the nation's economy. (If it performed according to expectations, the percentage of the economy under the aegis of the FMB should remain static, or even fall, over a period of time.)

Though the board would be shielded from day-to-day politics, it would be necessary to have a method for removing a board member for malfeasance in office. This could be done by a super majority vote of both houses of Congress, either two-thirds or three-fifths. As the Federal Reserve Board is charged with the task of adjusting interest rates to control inflation and enhance economic growth, the Federal Medicare Board's mission would be to insure that all Americans were provided with quality health care in a cost-effective manner.

A number of prominent Americans, including economists and politicians, have previously suggested the formation of a Federal Health Board to play a major role in the health care system. These include former senator Tom Daschle (who had been nominated to be the Secretary of Health and Human Services, but withdrew over tax issues), a Democrat from South Dakota, who has a special interest in health care reform and wrote a book about it called *Critical*,[15] as well as former senator Chuck Hagel, a Republican from Nebraska, Senator Max Baucus, a Democrat from Montana (who is Chairman of the Senate Finance Committee), and Ben Bernanke, the Chairman of the Federal Reserve Board.[16] However, various proponents of a Federal Health Board have different visions of its make-up and how it would function.

As managing the U.S. health care system would be a gargantuan task, the Federal Medicare Board would have a number of standing advisory committees to help the Board meet its mandates. These would include groups to deal with organizational matters, hospitals, therapeutics, diagnostics, provider and employee reimbursement and salaries, preventive medicine, oversight, and so forth. The committees would be composed of experts in each area chosen by the FMB and would be chaired by members of the FMB. The size of the committees would be decided by the FMB, with additional subcommittees formed to handle specific tasks. The latter might be transient if charged with analysis or solutions for particular problems, or permanent if the work were deemed to be on-going. Appointments and length of service for these subcommittees would be decided by the parent committees.

With new technology one of the drivers of health care spending, the Committee on Therapeutics and the Committee on Diagnostics, would play essential roles in vetting technological advances and reviewing current care to determine what Universal Medicare would cover. An article in the *Journal of the American Medical Association* (1999), by Dr. John M. Eisenberg of the Agency for Health Policy and Research, declared, "The goal of those who develop and provide medical technology and want to appeal to ... decision makers should be to provide value for money. The challenge ... is to create a health care system that recognizes value, rewards better outcomes, and encourages efficient use of limited resources."[17] Eisenberg went on to describe ten principles to consider when technology is being assessed. Another article by Perry and Thamer in the same issue of *JAMA* noted that "Health technology assessment (HTA) is the careful evaluation of a medical technology for evidence of its safety, efficacy, cost and cost-effectiveness and its ethical and legal implications, both in absolute terms and in comparison with other competing technologies."[18] They argue for the formation of a national-level agency to guide evaluation of medical technologies, including HTA studies when indicated. Under comprehensive health care reform, the Committees on Therapeutics and Diagnostics would assume that function. (According to a projection from the Congressional Budget Office, half of the increase in health care costs over the next 16 years will come from the use of new drugs and devices.[19])

There are a number of ways health care agencies tried to control the growth of medical technology in the past, including rationing, regulation, budgetary constraints, managed care, and certificates of need. Universal Medicare would simply cut off payment for the use of unproven technology. The Committees on Therapeutics and Diagnostics would analyze all treatments and tests that were being used or being proposed, judging which of them were worthwhile for patient care and whether they were cost-effective. They would then decide which of these UM would cover. Though an emphasis would be placed on evidence-based medicine in determining the procedures and therapeutic options that would be paid for, physicians would have to be given some leeway to try new approaches, even employing medications off-label when there was some data to support their courses of action. (Many new treatments have evolved in this fashion, such as the use of antiepileptic medications for migraine control and some antihypertensive drugs to dampen tremors.)

Universal Medicare would probably have to fund studies of some of the new technologies and therapies to determine their benefits. Some older treatments of uncertain value might also be subjected to controlled studies. (Questions have already been asked about aspects of medical care that have been endorsed for decades—such as performing routine annual physicals on young people, or routine chest x-rays in nonsmokers—wondering whether they are worthwhile. These services take time and expend resources that could be directed in a more productive fashion, including preventive care. A Commonwealth Fund report on achieving value in health care in 2007 estimated that $368 billion could be saved over 10 years with improved information and decision-making about the "relative clinical and cost-effectiveness of alternative treatment options."[20] The fiscal stimulus package championed by the Obama administration that became law in February 2009 included $1.1 billion for research on the comparative effectiveness of various drugs, medical devices, surgical procedures, and other treatments.)

The Committee on Therapeutics would also address questions of great sensitivity to many people when considering end-of-life care and futile care. (This is another reason to eliminate political influence from the health care equation.) Decisions in terms of treatment would be made on the basis of effectiveness and cost/benefit ratios and outside the political arena. No country can afford unlimited care for everyone for every condition. Undoubtedly, there would be people who would be unhappy with any restrictions that were imposed. But those who desired maximum therapy for everything, whether or not it was shown to be effective, could purchase Tier 3 insurance coverage to obtain the care they wanted (though not everyone would be able to afford it). Society's health care dollar would be aimed at therapies that worked and situations where improvement or recovery was possible.

Cost/benefit ratios might also have to be employed by the Committee on Therapeutics when deciding whether to authorize expensive treatments that might extend life for brief periods or minimally improve the quality of life in patients who were not terminal. Included would be treatments with biopharmaceutical agents that can increase survival in some cancers by several months and cost up to $100,000 for each year of use. Providing dialysis or various invasive procedures for people with severe dementia would also be policies to be reassessed.

Among the issues the Committee on Diagnostics would have to examine would be whether payments should be approved for screening cardiac CT scans, each of which runs to thousands of dollars and whose value is uncertain. (The cardiologists who own these machines refer their patients for the procedures and reap the financial rewards.) Should screening lung CT scans be done routinely on patients who are or were smokers? If so, how often? Since it would be working with a fixed budget (to be discussed later), the FMB and its committees would be forced to make hard decisions about where money should be spent, as it would not have unlimited resources at its disposal. There are lots of questions in all of these areas that need to be answered after careful analysis and deliberation. And those making these decisions must be shielded from pressure by politicians or special interests who want a particular path to be followed (as well as from possible liability suits or legal hassles). Of course, for those with Tier 3 coverage these questions would be moot.

The Committee on Therapeutics would also be allowed to negotiate prices for drugs with the pharmaceutical companies as an agent for Universal Medicare. (As previously noted, Medicare was prohibited from doing this when Part D was enacted in 2003. This was because Congress was guided in developing the bill by pharmaceutical industry lobbyists. And the coauthor of the measure, Congressman Billy Tauzin, the chairman of the House Commerce Committee, subsequently became a lobbyist for the drug industry. Attempts to change this regulation were blocked by Republicans in the Senate,[21] but will probably be enacted by the new administration.) Having exceptional purchasing power, the Committee would be able to lower prices, particularly if there were companies with competing products, ensuring major savings for the health care system and patients. (Estimated savings for current Medicare alone, if drug prices could be negotiated, is $43 billion over 10 years.[22]) Brand-name drugs and generics would all be in the mix, with efficacy and price determining which medications were preferred by the FMB (as advised by the Committee). Other drugs besides the preferred medications could be prescribed by physicians and used by patients. However, in some instances physicians would have to justify their use (allergy, or adverse response to preferred product, or ineffectiveness). If a patient simply wanted a nonpreferred medication or brand-name drug, he or she would have to pay for it, perhaps through Tier 3 coverage.

The Committee on Hospitals would determine the need for hospital beds in different cities and regions, the type of hospitals that were required, and the kinds of alliances among hospitals that might be useful in eliminating redundant services and reducing costs without negatively affecting care. It would work in concert with the regional entities that were responsible for the delivery of health care (to be discussed later). Their deliberations would have to be free of political interference from elected officials trying to preserve hospital beds in their districts. (The problem would be similar to the controversy regarding the closing of military bases, though on a smaller scale. The Committee on Hospitals would have the same role as the independent commission that was established to evaluate the viability of the bases.) Hospitals today are autonomous units run by universities, community boards, religious organizations, for-profit corporations, and so forth. Universal Medicare would not force any institution to close, even if it were deemed unnecessary or of poor quality, but would cut off its funding and stop paying for the maintenance of excess beds. Hospital executives would not be happy to have their fate in the Committee's hands, but regionalization of care could save considerable amounts of money for UM. (Perhaps some of the hospitals that lost funding could survive by serving Tier 3 patients, but this strategy would not save many of them.) The Committee would also decide if additional hospital beds or even new hospitals were needed in particular areas, perhaps because of population growth or poor quality of the existing institutions.

The Committee would work to enhance the quality of all U.S. hospitals, using financial incentives and disincentives to ensure that best practices were being followed and the necessary corrective measures were being taken. These efforts would be coordinated with the regional entities. In addition, decisions would have to be made about which institutions should have house staff and receive extra funding for the training of interns, residents, and fellows. Though house staffs improve patient care at hospitals, not all institutions are able to provide adequate teaching of these young physicians while utilizing their labor.

The responsibility for ensuring that prevention was integrated into Universal Medicare's planning, and then executed properly, would be under the aegis of the Committee on Preventive Medicine. Preventive medicine and health promotion would play important roles in fulfilling UM's mission. Premium health care requires prevention to be front and center, both for acute and chronic illnesses. This can mean longer survival for patients, with a better quality of life. It would also mean cost savings if there were fewer diabetics to treat because of preventive measures, or if high blood pressure were controlled and there were fewer strokes. Indeed, there are numerous ways that prevention and health promotion could help patients while saving health care dollars. There have been estimates that preventable conditions comprise about 70 percent of the total burden of illness and the related costs, with lifetime medical expenditures clearly connected to health behavior.[23] (As an example, the lifetime costs for smokers are about a third higher than for nonsmokers, despite the fact that their lives are shorter.[24])

In addition to working with established patients, more aggressive medical outreach programs are needed to bring people with chronic illnesses, or those prone to develop them, into the health care system. The earlier this is done, the better it will be, in terms of prevention and ultimate outcome. E-mails and phone contacts to keep tabs on patients with chronic illnesses and in prevention programs should also be used more frequently. (The 2007 Commonwealth Fund report estimated that effective national and state programs to reduce obesity could alone save $283 billion over 10 years.[25])

The Committee on Oversight and the Committee on Administration and Organizational Matters will be essential to Universal Medicare's success. The Committee on Oversight will work with an Inspector General's office to minimize the amount of fraud and corruption. Unfortunately, over the years since its inception, the Medicare program has been rife with fraud, with billions of taxpayer dollars lost. The problem has been a lack of proper monitoring, with providers upcoding or billing for patients never seen, hospitals being paid for unnecessary procedures or bills that were augmented by false coding, medical equipment makers billing and being paid for equipment that was not ordered, and so forth. There has never been enough oversight to prevent this type of behavior, and punishment was not severe enough when lawbreakers were caught. The Medicare employees who missed or did not aggressively pursue fraud and corruption on their watch were also not held accountable. Many of these government workers were simply content to pass the fraudulent costs on to the U.S. taxpayer. This type of behavior will not be tolerated in Universal Medicare, which will operate as a quasiprivate entity, able to discipline employees appropriately for poor performance.

Some corrupt, or at least anticompetitive, behavior has also been fostered by political interference in Medicare functions. As mentioned previously, when medical equipment makers were found to be billing excessively for various types of equipment, competitive bidding was instituted by Medicare to lower costs. Then, at the behest of lobbyists for the involved companies, Congress stepped in and pressured Medicare to reverse its actions, and the program continued to overpay for the equipment. This is one of the reasons why politics must be eliminated from all facets of UM's operations.

The Committee on Administration and Organizational Matters will be responsible for streamlining the various organizational and administrative functions of Universal Medicare. A corporate structure with appropriate sections to handle different operations and to establish clear lines of command is imperative in the new organization. Interactions with all the providers and health care facilities must also be simplified as much as possible. As noted, administrative and overhead costs now consume approximately 20 percent (or more) of the U.S. health care dollar, and this must be cut at least in half with health care reform. The savings of over $200 billion could cover a considerable portion, if not all, of the increased expenditures that will be required for universal access to care. (The single-payer system alone is a major step on the road to reduced administrative spending.) Medicare has been shown to be very efficient from an administrative standpoint, and there is no reason why this efficiency should not be transferable to Universal Medicare. In fact, it may be possible to design it to be even more productive, with even greater savings realized.

Proper provider reimbursement will, of course, be critical to controlling costs in a new health care reform program, with the decisions made by the Committee on Provider Reimbursement and Salaries. These include payments for services to hospitals, rehabilitation centers, imaging units, and other health care facilities, as well as to physicians and nonphysician practitioners (nurse practitioners, physician assistants, midwives). However, many of these medical personnel, in addition to RNs and physical therapists, will be paid directly by the institutions for which they are working. (Physician reimbursement will be discussed shortly.) Though the hospitals and the various health care facilities must be paid enough for their services to allow them to continue to operate with a small profit, costs must still be constrained and payments must not be excessive. Perhaps having competitive bidding for particular services among nearby hospitals and other entities might be a way to hold down costs, with patients being directed to the low-cost providers (as long as quality was comparable).

Executives and administrative employees of Universal Medicare must be paid competitively with government agencies and the private sector. But they cannot be given the generous bonuses and total compensation that top corporate executives have received independent of their job performances. Merit bonuses for personnel, however, should certainly be considered to enhance productivity. It will be up to the Reimbursement Committee to decide on the compensation for UM's executives and the various classifications of employees, with ratification necessary by the full FMB. The Committee will try, of course, for a Goldilocks solution: neither too high, nor too low, but just right, allowing Universal Medicare to attract competent personnel.

(In addition to the Federal Medicare Board, it should be helpful to divide the country into ten or twelve medical districts with twenty to forty million people each and to appoint District Medicare Boards to help administer the programs in conjunction with the FMB. They could focus more on local and regional issues with policy set from above.)

## Funding Universal Medicare

Current sources of funding for health care in the United States are shown in Figure 6.1. Universal Medicare will collect funds from contributors to the system and disburse them to providers (through administrative intermediaries). There are six potential sources of funding for Universal Medicare, the amounts and percentages of which would be spelled out in the enabling legislation. Since UM is a quasi-governmental, quasiprivate entity, it would not have the power to increase (or decrease) the funds it received and would instead have to approach Congress for any additional sums that were necessary for its operation. However, requests for

# Funding of U.S. Health Care

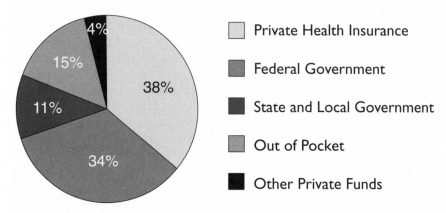

**Figure 6.1** Sources of funding for U.S. health care. Source: Center for Medicare and Medicaid Services, Office of the Actuary, National Health Statistics Group, National Health Expenditures Accounts.

supplementary funding would essentially be an admission of failure by UM, showing that its attempts to hold health care spending in check were not working. The six sources of Universal Medicare's operating funds would be the following:

1. Premiums from enrollees. As is the case with the current Medicare program, enrollees would pay a premium to obtain coverage. Every American would be eligible to participate, which means that many young, healthy individuals would sign up. These enrollees would be less likely to require expensive medical services and their premiums would help to subsidize the costs of those who were ill. As mentioned, UM enrollment would not be mandated initially, allowing Americans freedom of choice. But given the other sources of funding for the program, premiums would be kept low enough to make Universal Medicare a good value for anyone seeking health care coverage. The amount of these premiums would be determined by Congress with an automatic increase pegged to the rate of inflation. If the Federal Medicare Board wanted to raise the premiums for any reason, they would have to go to Congress for authorization. (To simplify the payments of premiums, arrangements could be made to have them deducted at work from employees' salaries and deposited automatically in Universal Medicare accounts. They could also be deducted automatically by the government from Social Security payments for seniors, or withdrawn monthly from people's bank accounts if participants so desired.)

2. The Medicare tax now in place. At present, there is a Medicare tax of 2.9 percent of wages, of which 1.45 percent is paid by the employer, and 1.45 percent is paid by the employee and withheld by the employer. The Universal Medicare tax would continue at the same rate for employees, but would be raised for employers as described below. Those who are self-employed would continue to pay the same 2.9 percent they currently pay. (If over time health care costs were held in check, the employees' portion of the tax could be reduced or even discarded completely.)

3. Universal Medicare employer tax/fee. Virtually every large business and many small businesses are now saddled with the task of paying for their employees' health care, either by purchasing coverage from insurance companies or self-insuring. In addition to the costs of the insurance, expenditures are required for administering these programs. Universal Medicare would eliminate the spending related to insurance and administration, saving these companies huge sums of money, as well as extricating them from having to deal with rising costs. And the legacy health care costs for their former employees would be taken off the books for many businesses, canceling future liabilities for the care of these retirees and generating further savings for them. The bulk of the combined business savings would be used to help fund the Universal Medicare program through a tax/fee. (It would be more of a fee than a tax, since it would come mainly from the money companies would save on their current health care, rather than cutting into their income or profits.) The hassles associated with health care would also be shifted away from businesses, allowing them to concentrate on their core functions.

The amount of the tax/fee that companies would pay Universal Medicare would have to be decided by Congress and might depend on the number of employees the businesses had, with an extra amount added for those with legacy costs. Over time, the tax/fees would equalize and would be determined by the number of employees alone, as no new legacy costs would be generated and the old ones would be winding down. Again, increases in the tax/fee would be pegged to the inflation rate, with any further increments subject to Congressional approval. Large corporations should welcome this type of trade-off to rid themselves of their health care burdens. It would also level the playing field to some extent between foreign companies that have operated in the United States in recent decades with no legacy costs and their old-line U.S. competitors, since all companies would have to pay into the system.

A problem arises, however, with those small businesses that don't currently provide health coverage for their employees. Some of them may not be generating enough income to pay for insurance, and adding a new tax/fee could make it hard for them to operate. Perhaps these companies could pay UM a lower amount, with the per employee tax/fee less for smaller companies with fewer employees. The details of how the tax/fees would be structured would have to be examined and resolved by Congress.

(Physicians for a National Health Program estimate that a 7 percent payroll tax on employers would be necessary to fund a universal health care program.[26] They also estimate that large businesses that provide health insurance for their employees currently pay about 8.5 percent for this benefit and would likely save money.)

4. Contributions from states. Medicaid, is a joint federal-state health program for the poor. The costs are currently shared by both the federal and state governments, with state funding responsible for a significant share. The amount varies by state, as each one decides independently how much it will spend on its program. Federal funds for Medicaid are channeled into each state based on a matching formula. States spent about $112 billion on Medicaid in 2004, with $176 billion coming from the federal government.[27] (State allocations for Medicaid were undoubtedly much higher by 2008.) If Medicaid were absorbed into Universal Medicare, states would save many billions of dollars, both in paying for health care services and administering the programs. A large part of this found money should be contributed to support Universal Medicare, the exact percentage being spelled out by Congress and indexed for inflation. Hopefully, the states that currently spend more money on health care for their poor residents would not be penalized by Congress because they were more compassionate, and some sort of equalizing formula would be devised. (State savings from ending the SCHIP program would also be contributed to UM.)

5. Deductibles and co-pays from patients. Any reform plan must take the issue of moral hazard into account (the consideration that an individual not subject to a risk will act differently than someone who has full exposure to that risk. In other words, a person not endangered by the full consequences of his or her behavior may act less carefully than he or she might if completely culpable for his or her actions.). Thus, to be certain that people do not overuse a free system of care, they should be responsible for a portion of the payments for the services they utilize, secured by a schedule of co-pays and deductibles. Since it is known that those less affluent are often unable to afford the deductibles and co-pays (which makes them reluctant to see physicians when they have a problem), the deductibles and co-pays could be indexed in some way to income. That would be more equitable and make it more likely that poor and middle class patients would go to the doctor early in the course of their illnesses. But even a small payment from those below the poverty line should be required in an attempt to prevent abuses. (Studies have shown no significant difference in health status between enrollees in free and cost-sharing insurance plans, though the former may use medical resources more often because of less out-of-pocket costs.[28,29])

Establishing standard deductibles and co-pays are fairly arbitrary; the intent is try to discover what amount will discourage unnecessary use of medical services but not deter people from visiting doctors when they are sick. These numbers can be determined by experts and set by Congress depending on the recommendations. Once the numbers are inaugurated, they can subsequently be adjusted by the FMB (if Congress grants them this discretion) depending on how medical care has been affected. For example, patients might be obligated to directly pay the first $1,000 of medical expenses annually, along with 20 percent of the next $5,000 ($1,000), and 10 percent of the next $5,000 ($500). Thus, patients would be responsible for a maximum of $2,500 of their medical expenses each year, including medications. The maximum expenditures per family could be set at $5,000. From these points on, Universal Medicare would cover all services fully. If overuse of services were found to be occurring at these levels of co-pays and deductibles, they could be ratcheted higher by the FMB. If patients were delaying seeing physicians and were failing to obtain appropriate care, the amount set for co-pays and deductibles could be reduced. These levels would also be decreased on a sliding scale for those of lower income.

(Another concept that might be considered is having a separate deductible for each episode of illness, rather than on a yearly basis. This would be similar to the way auto collision insurance is handled. Obviously, the deductibles would be set lower and UM would not make patients pay more for treating the same illnesses over two or more enrollment periods. If this were structured correctly, it might be fairer than other proposed deductibles and could encourage patients to continue to obtain care for specific problems. The parameters of this would have to be worked out to see if it was a viable alternative.)

In some other countries that have universal coverage, patients pay nothing or very little for medical care, which has resulted in overuse of services at times. Increasing the employer's tax/fee, or the government's contribution to Universal Medicare, could allow patients' co-pays and deductibles to be reduced or eliminated. But since the United States has not had any experience with universal access, it would probably be better to start with the co-pays and deductibles in place as restraints on unnecessary utilization, lowering them in the future if it were warranted. Some experimenting will be required to find the most efficient and effective way to promote appropriate care. (Physicians for a National Health Program suggest a 2 percent income tax from everyone to support universal health care, with the elimination of all out-of-pocket costs.[30] They estimate that it would be less than what people now pay for insurance costs, co-pays, and deductibles. However, it does not take moral hazard into account.)

6. Federal government funding. As noted, the federal government already pays for a large percentage of U.S. health care with the funds coming from general tax revenues or through tax subsidies. (Analysts have shown that Washington is currently responsible for about 60 percent of the nation's health care bill.) Included under funds from general revenues are its contributions to the Medicaid and SCHIP programs, its funding of the Veterans' Administration network, and its payments for Medicare Part B, C, and D. With employer-based health insurance premiums not being taxed, the federal government provides subsidies for this type of health coverage. If Universal Medicare was established through comprehensive reform, government spending on health care would remain level or even decrease over time, but all the funding would be directed to Universal Medicare.

In one way or another the payments for the cost of health care, no matter what form they may take, are ultimately borne by all citizens. If employers pay for health care, workers are given lower wages and fewer benefits in other areas, while the government loses tax revenues. If people are uninsured and need care, the cost of their services is included in the bills everyone else

**Table 6.1  Funding Sources for Universal Medicare**

| | |
|---|---|
| **1. Premiums from enrollees** | Amount determined by Congress |
| **2. Medicare tax** | Rate currently in place:<br>• 1.45% per employee<br>• 2.9% for self-employed |
| **3. Employer tax fee** | Pegged to number of employees and legacy costs.<br>Should be comparable to current health care spending by businesses, with special considerations for small businesses. |
| **4. Contributions from states** | Money saved by elimination of Medicaid and SCHIP programs would go to fund Universal Medicare. |
| **5. Deductibles and co-pays from enrollees** | Out-of-pocket payments currently 15% of health care expenditures—estimated $315 billion in 2008.<br>Out of pocket costs–would probably be less under Universal Medicare. |
| **6. Government contributions** | Federal government already pays for health care costs out of general tax revenues, contributions to Medicaid, SCHIP, VA, and payments for Medicare Part B and Part D.<br>Federal government also subsidizes employer-based health insurance, as premiums are not taxed.<br>Estimates of government portion of current health care show costs are about 60%.<br>Government spending on health care would remain level with Universal Medicare or decrease over time. |

receives, resulting in higher insurance premiums and higher taxes. And, of course, if the government pays directly for health care, taxes increase.

(A controversial issue that should be considered as part of health care reform is whether individuals whose life styles increase their risk of expensive, chronic illnesses should bear some responsibility for the cost of care, perhaps by having higher premiums, co-pays, and deductibles. This would include smokers, alcoholics, drug users, obese, and sedentary individuals, motorcyclists, and so forth. The problem here is that increasing their fees might stop them from seeking medical care, perhaps making it more difficult to treat them and driving costs up later. On the other hand, the way they live costs everyone else money to care for them at some point. Life insurance reflects these risks with higher rates for smokers, and there are higher premiums for motorcyclists, drivers with DUI convictions, and so forth. Would increasing their premiums, co-pays, and deductibles be added incentives to induce them to change their life styles? If they did change, the higher charges could be reduced. But it is unclear what approach should be taken.)

### Living Wills

All enrollees in Universal Medicare should be required to have living wills and advanced directives to reduce aggressive end-of-life care and futile care. The enrollment process for UM should include the registration of these documents and helping people to find the right formula for themselves. Besides saving Universal Medicare money, it would allow men and women to have their wishes observed and to be able to die with dignity. Individuals who wanted every option for care to be pursued, whether or not it was futile or of unproven value, could obtain Tier 3 coverage.

## Fixed Budget

Universal Medicare will be responsible for paying physicians, hospitals and all the other providers that furnish health care services for the plan's enrollees, as well as its own personnel and overhead. For this, a fixed annual budget that encompasses UM's total spending will be established by Congress that UM will have to adhere to; it is a simple method of restraining rising costs. The budget could be set as a percentage of the GDP and kept at that level, perhaps rising each year as the GDP did, but the percentage remaining the same. Sixteen percent of the GDP could be used initially, as that is what health care spending currently consumes. If Universal Medicare were able to eliminate a meaningful portion of the unnecessary medical services, fraud, waste, and administrative costs that currently plague the health care system, it could easily be able to live within its budget, even with the millions of uninsured who would begin receiving coverage.

As a reminder, unnecessary care is calculated to be 20–30 percent of current health care expenditures. With a total of $2.1 trillion estimated to be spent on health care in 2008, that comes to $420 billion squandered at the low end. Administrative costs are thought to be 15–25 percent of health care costs. Assuming it is 20 percent means that another $420 billion is being consumed here. Fraud takes another $50 to $100 billion. And there is also defensive medicine and futile care devouring the health care dollar (probably under the heading of unnecessary care). If one-third of the $900 billion plus that is misused could be saved, there would be more than enough money to care for the uninsured and remain within budget. Greater savings could be returned to the government, used to give bonuses to personnel, or to expand services such as preventive care. Some of it might also be kept as a "rainy day fund" in case the budget was exceeded in the future. However, if the expected savings were not realized, it would necessitate cutting back on some services.

If it appeared that the budget was going to be exceeded, the FMB, with the advice of its committees, would have to make decisions about which services would be reduced, taking into consideration their cost/benefits ratios. To some analysts, the use of cost/benefit ratios to determine services is a form of rationing. To others, it simply means making choices in a logical fashion when resources are limited. Whatever it is called, it must be employed if funding is lacking to pay for previously covered services. Unconstrained growth of health care spending is simply not an option, and Universal Medicare must function within its budgetary boundaries. But given the potential savings waiting to be harvested, it is likely that services will never have to be decreased if UM aggressively reins in unnecessary care and overhead.

Interestingly, as was noted in a recent article, spending on health care by various nations above a certain level (approximately $2,000 per capita) does not result in a significant improvement in health outcomes.[31] Nor does it heighten satisfaction with the health care system. Though the United States now spends more per capita than any other country on health care, its patients, physicians, hospital executives, and most citizens are less enamored with the performance of their system than the same groups in other developed nations. And in various regions in the United States, a study showed no correlation with the per capita expenditures on health care and the perception by patients of the quality of the care they received, even when there was a great variation in the intensity of services.[32] The above data suggests that budgeting for Universal Medicare should not diminish patient satisfaction with care or overall health outcomes.

(While health care spending in the United States has been skyrocketing disproportionate to the expansion of the economy in recent decades, no administration has placed restraints on federal funding for health care, thereby allowing Medicare and Medicaid to almost grow at will. Tying growth in health care expenditures to growth in the GDP would have been a sensible approach, but was not pursued. Having a fixed budget for Universal Medicare as a percentage of the GDP will automatically bring unfettered spending on health care back to earth.)

## Placing Physicians on Salary

Compensating physicians for the care they provide is a contentious issue, both in how payment is rendered (fee for service, capitation, salary) and the differences in income among the various fields of medicine. Because doctors generate a major portion of the demand for their own services,[33] if health care costs are to be brought under control, it is imperative that physicians' financial incentives to provide patients with more care, do more procedures, and order more tests be eliminated. Human nature cannot be changed, and so the mechanism for payment must be changed. Laurence Kotlikoff has noted that "The fee-for-service payment system is the primary contributing factor to the excessive Medicare and Medicaid growth. It has put spending on these programs largely on autopilot. . . . the government has positioned itself to be responsible for paying whatever the health care delivery system and the Medicare and Medicaid participants using the system collectively decide they want to provide and receive in terms of healthcare services."[34] This mechanism of payment cannot continue without eventually bankrupting the programs and severely damaging the remainder of the economy.

The estimate of unnecessary care, representing 20 to 30 percent of health care costs, is directly related to how physicians generate income, which is an expected consequence. The more they do, the more they receive. This may be a fine way to pay salesmen who sell couches or cars, but it is not the way a quality health care system should work. The only way to significantly reduce unnecessary and excessive care is to stop compensating physicians for piecework and pay them a salary, scrapping the incentives they have to provide more services. Undoubtedly, this idea will send up an immediate hue and cry from many physicians and organized medicine, as they would suddenly be facing an earth-shattering change. (However, even in the current system, about one-third of all physicians are salaried employees, with the percentage continuing to grow according to the AMA.[35])

U.S. physicians, historically, have been independent practitioners and individualists who were reluctant to submit to authority, although a large number now practice in groups. The concept of being on salary and no longer being paid for each service will require a cultural transformation and different mind-set for many physicians. But it must be done to control costs. (Intrusive monitoring of all physicians' services could theoretically reduce unnecessary procedures and other excessive care, but in practice would not work. It would be much too costly, requiring too many sophisticated monitors who were conversant with medical terminology, who understood the accepted rationales for surgery, procedures, and other services in various situations, and who were knowledgeable about the medical literature. And even if these people were available, physicians would still be able to justify unnecessary services with misleading reports. Placing doctors on salary which would abolish the incentives for excessive care, is the only way to change physician behavior.)

In addition to reducing unnecessary care, having physicians on salary would stop fraudulent billing. There would be no reason for physicians to upcode their bills for services or bill for fictitious care since doing so would not increase their income. Doctors would also no longer have to defend their use of what they consider appropriate coding for patient services when insurance companies or Medicare disagreed with them. And there would be no more attempts to game the system, as it would not bring greater remuneration. The amount lost to billing irregularities is difficult to discern, as accurate monitoring is impossible, but it is probably considerable. Putting physicians on salary would produce further savings for Universal Medicare if all the deceptive billing were eliminated.

(Some might say that having physicians on salary could serve as an incentive in a negative sense for them to avoid work, do fewer procedures, and provide fewer services, even when those services might be indicated. Physicians might also be less willing to render emergency care on nights and weekends. However, most individuals in the medical profession are properly motivated and have the drive to help people who are ill. In addition, there would be regional oversight bodies in place to monitor physicians' activities, guaranteeing that proper protocols were being followed and that the care was of high quality. Physicians who were significant outliers in procedures, with either too few or too many, would be watched carefully. Any doctor found to be careless or negligent could be punished by a reduction in salary, and, after repeated warnings, could be suspended from practice or lose his or her license. Small bonuses might also be given to those physicians who provided emergency care above a baseline level, just to add a minor monetary incentive to reward their efforts.)

Transforming the current payment methodology to having physicians on salary will be easier today than it would have been 20 years ago. This is because, as previously noted, over 30 percent of doctors already are salaried, working for hospitals, HMOs, or government agencies among other entities. Many of these physicians are quite content with their situations, receiving a paycheck without having to worry about running offices, hiring and managing personnel, collecting from patients and insurance companies, and so forth. They also have security and a better lifestyle. (Surveys have shown that salaried physicians are generally as satisfied with their work and income as their peers in private practice.[36]) Being compensated in this fashion is more in line with the way corporate executives are paid, rather than salespeople. As an incentive for improving care, physicians would also be given bonuses depending on how they performed on various parameters of quality (pay for performance) and on patient satisfaction surveys, as well as on the volume of patients seen. They would be rewarded for quality, performance, and productivity. (Quality of care landmarks for primary care physicians, surgeons, and some specialties have already been developed, but need to be further expanded. Patient satisfaction surveys could be filled out online once or twice a year and tallied by computer. Physicians who worked harder or longer hours and took care of more patients would be given bonuses for this, but there would not be the same incentive to inflate volume, as it would not be a major component of salary and would also be monitored.)

Even with physicians on salary it is important that their income levels be commensurate with the vital societal function they serve and the extra years of school and training needed to attain their positions. Because they get a late start in earning a living, it is important for them to be able to recover some of that lost income later on. They also work longer than average hours and are under great stress and pressure much of the time, literally responsible for life-and-death decisions. If the United States wants intelligent men and women to be their physicians, guiding their health care, and making the difficult decisions, they will have to pay them well. Even now the competition is fierce to attract the best students, with the legal profession, business, and the financial industry all making their pitches. And other areas of science beckon to them, pulling them away from medicine.

There is also the issue of the differential in income that now exists among the various fields of medicine because of the well-compensated procedures that some physicians perform and how that should affect their salaries in the future. As described previously, income levels can vary by hundreds of thousands of dollars, with certain specialties, such as orthopedics, ENT, neurosurgery, obstetrics and gynecology, cardiology, and gastroenterology, making considerably more money than primary care physicians. This differential is driven by the higher amounts insurance companies and Medicare pay for procedures, compared to the amounts for time spent interviewing and examining patients. (This is also an important factor related to unnecessary services.) When physician salaries are established, there will not be additional payments given for procedures and laboratory tests. These will be included in the compensation packages that are established.

Under Universal Medicare, the degree of the differential in income among the various medical fields will be reduced. There are several reasons why this is required. First of all, it is unfair. Physicians who have had equivalent amounts of training should not have widely divergent incomes because one performs surgery to alleviate a condition and the other prescribes medication to make someone better. There should not be a fixation on the greater value of surgery or procedures compared to cognitive work, and there should not be a major difference in salaries between procedure-oriented fields and those devoted to diagnosis and medical treatment.

There are a number of factors that should be taken into account in determining physicians' salary. These include the years of training, board certification, practice stresses (emergency call schedules, working under pressure for long periods, hospital responsibilities), difficulty of the work (intellectual and physical challenges), and experience (years in practice). The multiplier for experience might plateau after 15 or 20 years of practice and then decrease slightly after 25 or 30 years. Salaries would also be modified according to continuing education credits and board recertification at certain intervals—every five to seven years—as the best qualified physicians should be paid more. In addition, regional variations in the cost of living should be entered into the compensation formula, with doctors who work in more expensive locales paid more than those working in low-cost areas. There should be incentive bonuses as well, for physicians who are willing to practice in less popular locations, such as some inner city neighborhoods, rural towns, or Indian reservations.

Salaries should be pegged to the need for primary care physicians (PCPs) and to try and reduce the percentage of specialists coming out of training programs. From 1997 to 2005 there was a decline of 50 percent of U.S. medical graduates starting family practice residencies.[37] A recent survey of nearly 1,200 fourth-year medical students found that 23.2 percent expected to go into internal medicine.[38] However, only 2 percent were choosing careers in general internal medicine and becoming PCPs, with the others selecting better paying medical specialties. (More specialists means more procedures and therefore increased costs, but does not result in improved outcomes.[39]) Higher incomes alone are not the solution to the supply deficit, as working conditions and quality of life issues also play roles in the choice of medical fields. But if PCPs were paid appropriately for the important care they provide, it would match the respect and value that society places on their services, and more men and women would be likely to consider these fields. It is particularly important that enough PCPs be available to see patients, given the emphasis that Universal Medicare will place on preventive care and health promotion. (More general surgeons are also needed for trauma and emergency care, and their income levels should reflect that need.)

Though Universal Medicare will use specific criteria to determine salaries for practitioners in the various fields of medicine, professional societies will also be allowed to play a role. These bodies could negotiate with the Committee on Provider Reimbursement and Salaries to arrive at the final figures each year. (Professional societies would include groups such as the American Society of Internal Medicine, the American College of Surgeons, and the American Academy of Pediatrics. Smaller subspecialty groups would also be able to advocate their cause with the Committee.) The negotiations could be formalized with joint reviews by the Committee and the individual professional societies as part of the reimbursement process. A number of other countries already utilize this type of mechanism to decide how much physicians should be paid (as will be shown in the following chapter).

Physicians who are starting out in practice should adapt easily to being on salary since this was the way they were compensated during their training and they never experienced payments on the basis of fee-for-service. They will also never be faced with the expenses and hassles of setting up practices or paying buy-in fees to join group practices. As more senior physicians who are accustomed to the present system retire from medicine and new doctors take their place, it will seem as though having physicians on salary is the normal way of doing business.

Though physicians would be salaried as part of comprehensive reform, they would not be government employees subject to bureaucratic administrative control while they cared for patients. They could remain in their groups or individual practices and function as private contractors working for the regional entities, or they could take positions in group practices established by the regional entities and be employed directly by them.

(Alternative methods of eliminating physician incentives to generate services other than salary have also been proposed by some health care analysts. These include case-rate or episode-based payments, as is standard in U.S. hospitals; capitation, which has been generally unsuccessful when tried in the past; having a "medical home" for patients under the guidance of a primary care physician; and shared savings with primary care physicians as case managers.[40–42] All of these concepts are complex and would be difficult to implement across the board. Placing physicians on salary would be much simpler and would work better.)

Under Universal Medicare, hospitals would initially continue to be reimbursed based on a prospective payment system. They would be paid a predetermined amount related to the patients' diagnoses at discharge, with some adjustment for the higher costs in large urban areas. And to keep spending in check, there would be no reimbursement for avoidable complications that arose in the hospital, such as operative mistakes and certain types of infections, a policy that is now beginning to be instituted. In the future, other options for payment could be explored.

## Subsidized Medical Education

Another way to foster student interest in medicine is for the government or Universal Medicare to subsidize medical education. With the cost of medical school (tuition and living expenses) running over $60,000 per year in nonstate schools, physicians often graduate with hundreds of thousands of dollars in debt. (Physicians currently spend 9–12 percent of their income on school loans, with the prediction that this could rise as high as 31 percent by 2033.[43]) This can lead students to reject medicine out of hand, or when becoming doctors, to choose the more lucrative fields instead of primary care. If medical school were partially subsidized or paid for completely, more students might pursue medical careers and be drawn to primary care. This might be skewed even further if greater assistance were offered to those who went into primary care, with less dispensed to specialists. Additional subsidies for interns and residents who were being trained in primary care would be another incentive for them. If those who committed to primary care in medical school later chose a different field, they would be obligated to pay back the grants or subsidies they had received. And if physicians decided not to participate in Universal Medicare and but went into private practice outside the system instead, they would be responsible for the full cost of their medical educations. This would also pertain to physicians who became cosmetic surgeons on a fee-for-service basis.

## Regional Health Care Entities (RHEs)

Having physicians on salary, rather than being paid for each service, will change the structure of U.S. medicine. However, it would be difficult for Universal Medicare to administer all aspects of health care centrally, establishing and monitoring tens of thousands of practices, while paying every physician directly. Intermediaries will be required to do this on a regional level, with UM setting the standards that have to be followed and disbursing funds to the regional entities. These entities will be charged with organizing health care in their regions, paying salaries to the physicians, reimbursing hospitals, and other providers for their services. To increase efficiency, these regional bodies will each be given responsibility for the care of 1–5 million people, with the Federal Medicare Board choosing the organizations that will deliver medical services in each region. They could select from entities already in existence, such as medical schools, consortiums of hospitals, insurance companies, IPAs, or large physicians' groups, or they could encourage the formation of new entities to provide the health care in particular locations. Kaiser Permanente and similar multispecialty organizations would be prime candidates to be Universal Medicare's delegated health care managers. (Insurance companies currently act as third party administrators (TPAs) for businesses that are self-insured.[++] In this role, they service the plans, rather than profiting by assuming risk.)

Universal Medicare would sign agreements with these RHEs to manage health care in an area for three-year periods, renewable after two years if both parties were satisfied with the arrangements. These would be service contracts with established profit margins to eliminate incentives to withhold services or interfere with patient care. (This could be an opportunity for insurance companies to reinvent themselves and adapt to an environment in which comprehensive reform would drastically reduce their inflated salaries and earnings.) Whatever their configuration or origins, all of these entities would be working for Universal Medicare. They would contract with the physicians, hospitals, and other health care facilities in their area of responsibility, paying physicians' salaries and reimbursing other providers for their services. After a few years, when the volume of services generated became more predictable, these RHEs might require competitive bidding from hospitals and other medical facilities that wanted to provide patient services, signing up the low bidders as long as quality was maintained. (Over time, UM might also find that certain models of the RHEs were able to deliver the best care in a cost effective way and would give these organizations the new contracts.)

Though physicians would be salaried and essentially employees of the RHEs, they would retain some autonomy in that they could continue to maintain their offices along with their nursing and secretarial staffs, if they desired. They would be given extra money by Universal Medicare for the administrative costs of running their offices. Since there would be no interface with insurance companies about preapproval for tests and procedures, or haggling about coverage issues or over reimbursement, less staff would be required—a savings for the health care system. With economy of scale and with the RHEs behind them to negotiate prices, purchases of medical equipment and supplies would also be less expensive for physicians' offices, delivering additional savings. Eventually, in the name of productivity as well as to reduce costs, the RHEs might gather groups of physicians into dedicated medical buildings to serve their communities, closing many of the scattered, less efficient offices. In addition to primary care physicians, specialists would be readily available in these facilities to provide consultations and testing, along with radiology and out-patient surgery. However, primary care physicians' offices and Immediate Care facilities to serve the public would be located in all areas where the demographics made sense.

Even though physicians would be salaried under the new system, charges for the assumed value of their services would have to be posted in order to have patients pay the proper deductibles and co-pays. These would be collected by the physicians' office staffs and deposited in RHE accounts by electronic transfer. If the fees were not collected at the time of service for whatever reason (emergency care, hospitalization, lack of funds, etc.), the RHEs would bill the patients later for the amount owed. A running total of the UM status of every patient in terms of deductible and co-pays would be available in online accounts (separate from health information), accessible to the patient's RHE and to physicians' offices who knew the patient's password.

If comprehensive reform were enacted with physicians placed on salary, a transitional period of several years would be necessary to complete the switch, with continued fee-for-service during this interval. Payment during that time would probably be based on the current Medicare scale until the changeover was accomplished.

Alternative practitioners would not be covered under Universal Medicare, unless there was scientific evidence of benefit for their treatments. If patients wanted to consult or be treated by naturopaths or homeopaths, they would have to pay for the services out of pocket. Similarly, chiropractic therapy would not be reimbursed, aside from specific treatments shown to be of value in controlled studies. (Some low back pain appears to respond as well to chiropractic manipulation as to standard medical therapy, and that particular intervention would be paid for. However, frequent visits over a lengthy period of time, along with nutritional supplements and other treatments of unproven value, would not be reimbursed.)

## Electronic Health Records

A highly functional. integrated computer system interconnecting Universal Medicare with all physicians' offices, along with other providers and health care facilities, will be an essential part of comprehensive reform. Because of the fragmentation of the current health care system, much of the care given is not coordinated among the various physicians who attend a patient. Though Medicare patients on average obtain care from seven different physicians each year, these doctors are not linked together clinically, financially, administratively, or electronically.[45] This must change. The electronic connections envisioned under Universal Medicare would have two separate parts—patients' medical records and patients' financial information.

In terms of medical information, physicians would be required to keep electronic health records (EHRs) for all their patients that were updated each time the patient was seen or a test or procedure was performed. The records would be stored on the Internet (as well as on physicians' computers or servers) and would be accessible to any physician or provider who knew the patient's password, as well as to the RHEs. In addition to a narrative of the patient's history and physical examinations, a chronological flow sheet would be maintained of all the medications the patient had taken and for what conditions they had been given. This would include lists of any allergies, adverse effects, or interactions with other medications. Similar flow sheets would be kept of all tests that were performed. These inventories would result in considerable savings for the health care system, while protecting patients from needless injuries and delayed treatments. Unnecessary duplication of tests would be reduced, as well as therapy with medications that had previously failed or had caused significant side effects. All consultations and past data on every patient would be immediately available to the treating physicians, expediting diagnoses and treatment, and improving care while saving money. (Proper safeguards in terms of privacy would have to be carefully established and followed.)

Patients' health care financial records would be stored separately on the Internet and would be accessible to physicians and other providers who had the proper passwords, as well as to Universal Medicare personnel and the RHEs. This information would be kept current by physicians' offices and other health care providers. It would allow UM, the RHEs, and physicians' offices to make immediate adjustments in patients' obligations regarding premiums, co-pays, and deductibles, thus producing more accurate collections.

Electronic prescribing (ERx) is already being utilized in many physicians' offices, having been given a boost by the Medicare Modernization Act of 2003.[46] With ERx, physicians and their offices are able to transmit precise, readily understandable prescriptions electronically to pharmacies. This eliminates numerous mistakes, including those from illegible handwriting that can result in the wrong medications or wrong instructions being given, with potentially life-threatening consequences. Though ERx is still optional under Medicare, a number of health insurance plans and Medicare have provided financial incentives to physicians who are utilizing this technology. When ERx becomes mandatory along with the general use of electronic health records at some point in the future, patients' medication data will be immediately available to all prescribing physicians. This will minimize problematic drug interactions and duplicate orders from different doctors. Proper controls for handling narcotics and other dangerous drugs will also have to be adopted. In addition to increased safety and improved care, ERx should save money for the health care system.

The electronic interface among Universal Medicare, the RHEs, the participating physicians and other providers, regarding payment status and medical records, will be dependent on the computers and software that are employed. Communication must be easy and fast, with all the units compatible. Setting the system up will not be cheap, with hundreds of thousands to millions of terminals needed along with the necessary software. But for Universal Medicare to function effectively and efficiently, this electronic network is essential. Since all physicians and other providers will be required to have the proper computer terminals and be part of the system, UM should subsidize their purchase and maintenance. Though the initial outlay will be costly, long term savings should be substantial. With multiple companies vying for these lucrative contracts, reasonable prices for the equipment and maintenance should be attainable.

President Bush, in 2004, established a goal of having electronic health records for the vast majority of Americans by 2014, but success in this undertaking appears unlikely.[47] In July 2007, only 14 percent of doctors had basic EHR systems and only 4 percent had fully functional systems. High costs and minimal returns on investment were the major reasons for the low implementation of the technology, with an average price of $20,000 for each EHR unit. Many of the systems also did not work well for physicians with, what might be called, poor "operability." Another significant problem was the lack of "interoperability" between the different systems. Developing the proper software to overcome this failing should be a priority for Universal Medicare. The new initiative by President Obama as part of his economic stimulus package should accelerate the use of EHRs by more medical practices.

## Physician Extenders

The number of primary care physicians is currently insufficient to provide care for patients, instruct them in-depth about healthy living, and monitor those with chronic illnesses. This deficiency may become even more glaring with preventive care and health promotion expected to be an integral part of comprehensive health care reform. Incentives to attract more students into primary care medicine have already been discussed, but growth will take time, and the ultimate number may still fall short of what is needed. Another option that should be pursued is the increased use of physicians extenders—personnel who can serve some of the functions of physicians. These include physician assistants (PAs) and nurse practitioners (NPs; though social workers and pharmacists can also be utilized in some situations). Programs for PAs and NPs should be expanded and the education of individuals who elect to go into these fields should be subsidized.

Both PAs and NPs are midlevel practitioners who receive considerable clinical training before they are given responsibility for patients. They emerge from master's level programs, the nurses with prior RN or BSN degrees, the PAs from varied backgrounds including military medics, EMTs, nurses, lab, and radiology technicians. The PAs are given an abbreviated medical school curriculum with clinical rotations in the various medical fields. Most NPs already have years of clinical experience as nurses. There are some specialized residency programs for PAs, such as emergency medicine, surgery, and anesthesiology, but their practical knowledge also comes from preceptor training. (There are currently 125,000 nurse practitioners and 68,000 physician assistants in the United States.[48])

PAs and NPs can play effective roles both in delivering care for acute and chronic illnesses and in working with patients on prevention. (Studies have shown comparable outcomes by nurse practitioners and physicians for patients randomly assigned for treatment in an ambulatory care setting.[49]) Preventing diabetes, AIDS, coronary artery disease, cancer, and hypertension, among other conditions, is much more effective (and less costly) than dealing with these problems when they are full-blown and have a host of complications. If primary care physicians were too busy to spend enough time with patients to explain the actions necessary to forestall or effectively manage illnesses and the rationale behind life style changes, the education of these patients could be assumed by PAs and NPs. Patient care and/or instruction could take place in physicians' offices, community clinics, patients' homes, or other settings. (Health promotion programs in the workplace have been shown to be particularly effective.[50]) Physicians would provide back-up for the PAs and NPs if anything unexpected was encountered.

There are also certain procedures known to be vital preventive measures that are not being done frequently enough, either because patients are not attuned to the need for them, are worried about the expense, or there are not enough specialists to perform the studies. These would include mammography, pap smears, and colonoscopy. With universal access to care, and cost less of an obstacle for patients, along with increased education about prevention, the demand for these and other procedures will increase significantly, and there will not be enough specialists to meet the demand. There is no reason why PAs and NPs can not be trained to perform procedures such as colonoscopy with physicians in attendance, the latter perhaps supervising three or four of them at once and intervening when lesions are found or questions are raised. (There will be no opposition to this scenario by physicians because of financial considerations, since they are being paid a salary, rather than fees for each procedure.) This will allow many more colonoscopies to be performed and people screened for colon cancer. And if a patient is known to have a problem beforehand, a gastroenterologist or surgeon can always perform the procedure. Similarly, PAs and NPs can be trained to do other screening tests. (A number of state legislatures have recently been wrestling over bills to extend the scope of advanced nurses' practices, to allow them to substitute for physicians in instances where there are shortages.[51] There is concern, however, about the lack of uniformity among the states in defining the areas of responsibility for these nurses and limitations on the services they can provide.)

## Malpractice Reform

The comprehensive reform plan as described will lower overhead and administrative costs (single payer system), reduce unnecessary and excessive care (putting physicians on salary), and will bolster preventive care (better compensation for PCPs and more physician extenders). However, it also has to address the issues of medical negligence, malpractice, and defensive medicine—the latter also being responsible for unnecessary care. As shown previously, the current system does not work to curtail negligence or to reasonably indemnify those who have been injured. The entire system must be modified and made more equitable to physicians and injured patients, while finding ways to cut medical negligence. The role of liability attorneys and the method for compensating them must be changed as well.

If physicians believe a new system is fair and not stacked against them, they will be more willing to testify against their peers who have been guilty of malpractice and see them penalized, either financially or with sanctions. In addition, physicians need to know that they will be protected when there are maloccurrences, bad outcomes for patients that are not the physicians' fault, and that they will only be liable if they are negligent. And injured patients must be protected, and compensated fairly and promptly, by any new system that is devised.

Mandatory review of all claimed malpractice cases by panels of physicians (in the same field as the accused physician) would be a major step forward. The peer panel would decide in each case whether negligence had indeed occurred and whether there had been injury because of it. (These doctors would have the same training as the accused physician and would be knowledgeable about the standard of practice. They would be from different geographical locales than the accused physician and would not have known that person.) Plaintiff's attorneys and defense attorneys would still present their cases, but before this physicians' panel rather than a jury. It is assumed that arguments here would be based on factual evidence, with emotional entreaties omitted, and that cases would be adjudicated quickly. If the panel decided there had been negligence and injury, a judge who specialized in malpractice would decide the amount of money to be awarded. If either party were unhappy with the decision, they could appeal it to a three judge malpractice panel. If they were still dissatisfied with the judgment, they could then request a trial by jury. However, if the requesting party lost the case, he or she would be responsible for court costs and the winner's legal costs. Strict limits on noneconomic damages, such as pain and suffering, would also be part of the reform package, as this is a subjective perception that cannot be accurately measured to make a valid determination. (Plaintiffs' and defense lawyers could bypass the entire process if both parties agreed to a settlement before the case was presented to the physicians' panel.)

If, under comprehensive reform, plaintiff's lawyers continue to be compensated on a contingency basis for handling malpractice cases, they should be assessed a percentage of the court costs in losing cases when requesting a trial by jury, equal to the percentage they would have earned if they had won. They should also be required to offer clients in malpractice cases the option of being billed for services at an hourly rate.

(There have been suggestions that all medical injuries should be handled on a no-fault basis. While there are some advantages to this approach, it would not identify substandard physicians by ascertaining when negligence had occurred. In addition, if compensation were awarded for maloccurrences, which are inherent in many disease processes, it would become very expensive for the health care system.)

The method of dealing with malpractice cases as described above is fair and equitable to both physicians and patients. If instituted, it should be enough to significantly reduce defensive medicine, because physicians would know that if an action were brought against them, they would be judged by a panel of their peers who would understand the reasons for their conduct and would decide cases on the basis of the evidence. The cost of malpractice insurance would also drop precipitously with these reform measures. But rather than have salaried physicians pay its cost, it should be borne by Universal Medicare. This could be done through self-insurance or negotiated malpractice coverage with insurance companies, contracting with them for liability protection.

As noted previously, medical negligence causes unnecessary deaths and injuries and is a contributor to heightened health care costs. Two aspects of negligence have to be dealt with: systemic deficiencies and incompetent physicians. Reduction in systemic errors has to be driven by quality control measures, learning where and why mistakes occur, and then establishing rules to address those matters. Systemic problems are easier to spot and attack in a hospital setting where there already are standard operating procedures in place for most contingencies, and it is simple to issue directives for employees to follow (such as washing hands after touching patients to prevent infections). It is more difficult to ferret out mistakes in the community where there are many different offices and facilities with different codes of practice. E-prescribing should help control medication errors in the future, and electronic health records should reduce missteps because of oversights or insufficient data.

As part of reform, substandard and impaired physicians should also be handled by peer review panels of doctors (preferably from other geographical areas) who would be able to assess physicians' conduct and levels of competence. However, physicians forwarding complaints and those doing peer review to discipline doctors would have to be granted safe harbors through Congressional legislation, with protection from possible suits for slander or restraint of trade. If physicians were not protected from lawsuits, they would be unwilling to report negligence or incompetence, or to act in a disciplinary capacity. The peer review panels should be able to recommend suspension or removal of a physician's license to the state medical board, supervision for a defined period, and/or reeducation.

## Control of Fraud

It was stated previously that having physicians on salary would virtually eliminate them as a source of health care fraud. Removing insurance companies from the main arena of health care would also reduce their fraudulent and deceptive behavior. However, hospitals and other health care facilities, medical equipment, and device makers will all have to be evaluated to be certain their requests for payment are honest and accurate. Close oversight will be necessary, with competitive bidding for contracts wherever this is feasible. Electronic health records combined with proper software programs should make monitoring of every patient's tests and equipment easier, further decreasing fraud. There should also be more encouragement of whistle blowers by Universal Medicare, with the promise of appropriate rewards if large sums have been stolen. For those who commit fraud, civil financial penalties, as well as criminal actions, should be pursued vigorously.

## Physician Conflicts of Interest

Physician conflicts of interest regarding self-referral for procedures and services will end once physicians are on salary. However, other conflicts of interest, such as payment to physicians by drug companies or device makers to have them act as consultants or lecturers, must continue to be scrutinized. A number of medical schools and some hospitals have already instituted regulations that severely restrict relationships between staff physicians and outside entities. However, rather than outlaw them completely as some have proposed, the connections should be meticulously examined, since the companies in question may be useful for funding research or medical education, not all of which can be provided by Universal Medicare. Whether there is a quid pro quo has to be determined before concluding that a conflict of interest exists and should be terminated. It should be remembered that with physicians on salary under comprehensive reform, some of them may be looking for other sources of income, which could lead to actions that might be contrary to best medical practices and patient care. On the other hand, physician research activity should not be foreclosed because of a lack of funds. It is a fine line that UM and the RHEs may have to walk.

## Direct Consumer Advertising

Direct consumer advertising on radio, TV, the print media, and the Internet for prescription drugs, medical devices, and special tests raises health care costs and is an impediment to proper care. Though free speech issues may cause some problems, advertisements for medical products that are obtainable only under a physician's order should be banned from the general media. This prohibition might exclude lifestyle drugs such as Viagra and similar products, and cosmetic procedures such as Botox and liposuction. (But the latter would not be covered by Universal Medicare, and the former would probably receive limited coverage from the program.) It is unlikely that participating physicians in Universal Medicare would advertise, because they would accrue no benefits from generating increased tests or procedures. If cosmetic surgeons or private doctors who did not participate in Universal Medicare wanted to market themselves, there should be no objections.

Some aspects of what comprehensive reform is and isn't should be emphasized to allay public concern about a major program that will affect their daily lives. First of all, Universal Medicare is not "socialized medicine" and will not be run by the government. Though it will have government backing, it will be a wholly independent, private entity controlled by its own executive board, free of political or governmental interference. The Federal Medicare Board will establish overall policies for the organization, but health care will be managed by the regional entities. People's ability to use their own doctors will not be impacted. But since they will not be restricted by particular insurance plans, patients will actually have more freedom to choose the physicians they want. And doctors will be liberated to practice a higher quality of medicine. They will no longer have to worry about generating income with the services they provide and will not have to be concerned about defensive medicine. Comprehensive reform will correctly place patients and physicians at the center of the health care system, allowing them to make the right decisions about care without interference from the insurance companies.

**Table 6.2  Potential Savings from Comprehensive Health Care Reform**

1. **Unnecessary care**
   Estimates of 20–30% of health care costs (includes defensive medicine).
   $2.1 trillion overall expenditures.
   Low estimate of 20% places unnecessary care at $420 billion.
   Can cut at least 75% of unnecessary care by putting physicians on salary and ending defensive medicine through malpractice reform.
   **Savings: $315 billion**

2. **Administrative costs and overhead**
   (Includes costs of health insurance companies for both group and individual policies, costs of offices of physicians and other providers to interface with insurers, hospital costs to interface with insurers, costs for drugs and other services that are consumed by interface with insurers, Medicare, Medicaid, and other government health care costs used for administration.)
   Estimates of administrative costs range from 15–25% (some higher, some lower); if an average estimate of 20% is used for this category, the cost is placed at $420 billion.
   If 50% of this can be cut,
   **Savings: $210 billion**

3. **Fraud**
   (Includes corporate fraud, individual practitioners false billing, or upcoding.)
   Estimates in range of $50–100 billion dollars annually (could be low).
   Average of $75 billion.
   If 50% of this could be saved by having physicians on salary and better monitoring of providers through improved computer programs,
   **Savings: $37.5 billion**

4. **Drug costs**
   Currently, approximately 12.1% of health care costs, or $254 billion.
   Should be able to cut at least 20% of this by negotiating prices with drug companies and greater use of generics. Also, use of evidence-based medicine to determine whether or not high-cost drugs are beneficial.
   **Savings: $51 billion**

5. **Use of electronic health records**
   Some commentators have suggested savings in the realm of hundreds of billions of dollars with the use of EHRs. Would significantly decrease duplicate testing and treatments.
   **(Possible) Savings: $20–50 billion**

6. **Preventative medicine**
   Promoting healthy living and preventative care.
   Savings uncertain, but potentially very large.
   **(Possible) Savings: $50–100 billion**

**Table 6.2** *(Continued)*

**7. Decreasing medical negligence**

> Stringent quality control measures and malpractice reform could cut medical
>     negligence.
> Savings uncertain, depends of effectiveness of measures.
> **(Possible) Savings: $50 billion**

**Likely savings from comprehensive reform**

> $315 billion
> 210 billion
> 37.5 billion
> 51 billion
> $ 613.5 billion

**Possible additional savings**

> $50 billion
> 100 billion
> 50 billion
> $ 200 billion

No matter what happens in the short run, comprehensive health care reform will ultimately be enacted in the United States. The country cannot afford to disregard this program, given the explosion in health care costs and the growth of unfunded liabilities. It is just a question of when the realization of the need for it sinks in, and this is contingent on the political climate. Reform programs that are geared to the market and don't have stringent cost controls are recipes for failure. A single-payer system that places physicians on salary, removing their incentives for unnecessary services, is the least complex, most rational way to proceed. And the sooner it is in place, the better off the country will be. Other reform plans that seek to cut administrative costs and overhead without tackling physicians' financial conflicts of interest could partially lower costs, but both aspects are needed for a program to be fiscally sound. It is imperative that reform measures curtail the entrepreneurial behavior of physicians, if long-term costs are to be controlled.

The clock is ticking, and the United States' future financial obligations from Medicare and Medicaid keep rising and will saddle succeeding generations with back-breaking debt. This is in addition to the immediate effects of a bloated and inefficient health care system that many people can't afford, which delivers an uneven quality of care. Comprehensive reform will provide Americans with efficient, effective health care with built-in cost constraints. In addition, it will allow businesses to shed the burden of employee care and states to bury the problems and expenses of Medicaid. The United States must move forward.

There will be some complaints about a tiered system of care under comprehensive reform, with people saying it is not fair to allow more affluent individuals to have more options than those less wealthy. However, this situation now exists to an even greater degree. Those with more money get better care, whether they have better insurance policies or pay for services out-of-pocket. At least with comprehensive reform, and unlike the current system, everyone will have basic health care, with many of the Tier 3 options available to the wealthy being of questionable value. More elaborate and expensive care is not necessarily better care. And if people have money, they should be able to spend it the way they want, whether it is for larger homes, more expensive cars, or Tier 3 health care. The main goals of a reform program are to provide basic care for everyone and to constrain costs.

There will also be objections to implicit rationing with comprehensive reform, given that it is a program that provides care with a fixed budget. However, this is a more logical way to approach health care. No society can afford to pay for everything for everyone. If a point is reached where funds are running out during a particular fiscal year, decisions will need to be made about which services to cut, with cost/benefit ratios the main factor in the determination.

Having a government-supported entity running the U.S. health care system may sound like an outrageous idea to many people, particularly those who believe that market-based solutions are the answer to economic problems. However, a $700 billion bailout (or more) of the nation's financial system by the government would have also been considered outrageous by those same people only a short while ago. Additional recent actions by the government contrary to free market ideology include a rescue of the nation's largest insurance company, the takeover of Fannie Mae and Freddie Mac, financing the acquisition of a failing investment bank by another bank, and loans to the major automakers. Many of these maneuvers occurred under the aegis of a Republican administration with a conservative bent, reinforcing the concept that government intervention in the economy may sometimes be necessary when the alternatives to such actions are worse. And President Obama has followed this with an extraordinary economic stimulus package. Universal Medicare can be considered as a peremptory move by the government to save the health care system that is similar to the financial bailout. Though the health care crisis has evolved more slowly than the recent financial meltdown, the long-term ramifications for the economy may be just as dire. Restructuring the health care system in a way that can permanently constrain runaway costs, while providing universal access to care, must be adopted as soon as possible. The anticipated huge federal budget deficits in the next several years should not be seen as a reason for inaction. Comprehensive reform can save the nation money on health care costs and bolster the economy.

Comprehensive health care reform under Universal Medicare is not a perfect system. But it is better than any of the proposals being offered and will be able to meet the goals of universal access to care, with control of costs.

(The recent rise in unemployment is an added inducement to expedite comprehensive reform. With so much of health care coverage tied to employment, the number of the uninsured is bound to rise, leading to more deficiencies in care and more preventable deaths and disabilities.)

## CHAPTER 7

# PROPOSALS FOR U.S. HEALTH CARE REFORM AND A BRIEF SURVEY OF OTHER NATIONS' HEALTH CARE SYSTEMS

The more simple anything is, the less likely it is to be disordered, and the easier repaired when disordered.

—Thomas Paine, *Common Sense*[1]

Americans want major improvements in the health care system, as care grows increasingly expensive for those with and without insurance, and unaffordable for many. In addition, traversing the intricate labyrinth of insurance coverage to obtain approval for tests and treatments, to explain discrepancies, or to generate payments, is exceedingly difficult, even for those who have the time and expertise. Both liberals and conservatives, the unions and big business, acknowledge that the current arrangement is not working and that changes are needed,[2] though there is no consensus on the particulars of a program. But the dialogue has been ongoing through policy institutes and academic centers, by politicians and economists, in the popular media and scholarly journals. Thus, the proposal advanced in this book for comprehensive health care reform has not been generated in a vacuum.

A number of programs for reform have recently been offered and have received some traction and varying degrees of support, but they fail in different ways to meet the necessary criteria for success. As mentioned, no reform plan will work unless it is simple and straightforward, provides universal (or near-universal) access to care, and imposes realistic constraints on expenditures. Breaking the linkage between employment and health insurance with portability of coverage is also important. The two plans that have undergone the most scrutiny are those put forth by John McCain, when he was a presidential candidate, and President Barack Obama's. Given Obama's election with a Democratic majority in both houses of Congress, Obama's plan, or some variation of it, is likely to be enacted. But even with the modifications that are bound to occur as the plan wends its way through Congressional hearings and committee meetings, it will not have the crucial elements to make it successful.

Both the McCain and Obama plans rely, in varying degrees, on market-based solutions to reform health care, using the current players (the insurance companies) to provide coverage (the McCain program was much more market-driven). Senator McCain stated in an article in *The New England Journal of Medicine* in October 2008 that "Americans want a system of health care that allows everyone to afford and acquire the treatment and preventive care they need and the peace of mind that comes with knowing they are covered."[3] In an article in the same issue, Senator Obama said, "We need health care reform now. All Americans should have high-quality, affordable medical care that improves health and reduces the burdens on providers and families."[4] Both Senators McCain and Obama realized that health care reform is an urgent priority for Americans, but offered different visions of how to achieve that end.

## The McCain Health Care Plan

McCain's health care reform plan was actually the more radical of the two programs, based on a classical conservative philosophy that stresses individual responsibility and competition.[5] However, it potentially left more Americans uninsured. The central tenet of McCain's plan was an end to the tax exclusion given for the health insurance premiums paid by employers.[6] In other words, the cost of workers' health coverage, if provided by employers, would have been treated as income by the federal government and the employees would have had to pay taxes upon the amount of the premiums. This change was projected to raise about $3.6 trillion over a 10-year period.[7] The revenue generated by this strategy would have paid for refundable tax credits from the government of $2,500 for individuals and $5,000 for families who purchased private insurance in the open marketplace, or to partially offset the taxes if their employers provided the insurance. McCain's program would also have deregulated the insurance markets and allowed them to operate across state lines, which he and his economic advisors believed would have spurred competition and led to lower prices. (This claim has been questioned by analysts.[8] There are only a few major insurers left after a number of mergers and acquisitions. They share pricing and policy with each other and act almost like a monopoly.)

To be certain that coverage was available for all, McCain would have created a plan that guaranteed access through an insurance pool to those who were medically uninsurable in the market. Individually purchased policies would have been promoted, with less comprehensive, cheaper coverage encouraged, providing fewer benefits for enrollees. (These insurance plans would have been less expensive to purchase, but the policyholders would have been responsible for more of the costs of care.) In addition, Medicare payments would have been restructured with bundled compensation used for episodes of care and some payments made on the basis of outcomes. McCain also believed that liability reform was an important part of overall health care reform, and his plan would have required caps on medical malpractice suits.[9]

Aside from the bundling of Medicare payments for episodes of care, there were no substantive proposals as part of the McCain program to restrict unnecessary services in order to control spending. All the other measures envisioned to constrain costs were vague and nonspecific, and it is uncertain how much would have been saved if they were all instituted.

Though the move to de-couple health insurance from employment was arguably a move in the right direction, the method used of eliminating the current tax benefits could have resulted in higher taxes for many Americans. In addition, more Americans could have been pushed into the ranks of the uninsured as their employers dropped coverage and they were unable to afford insurance, even with the refundable tax credit that was given.

An article in the journal *Health Affairs* in September 2008 analyzing the McCain health reform plan noted that "The decline of job-based coverage would force millions of Americans into the weakest segment of the private insurance system—the nongroup market—where cost sharing is high and covered services are limited. Senator McCain's proposal to deregulate this market would mean that people in it would lose protections they now have. These changes would diminish the security of coverage for most Americans, especially those who are not—or someday will not be—in perfect health."[10] The McCain program would have been most beneficial for the young and the healthy, who could have used their tax credits to purchase cheaper insurance in the private marketplace.[11]

Administrative costs would undoubtedly have ballooned if McCain's plan had been put into effect. Its reliance on the individual insurance market involved much greater underwriting than large group policies to determine what each person should pay for coverage, depending on his or her state of health, age, and other factors. The guaranteed access for all Americans, notwithstanding illnesses or preexisting conditions, would also have been costly to administer in conjunction with existing state high-risk pools. (Administrative costs for individual policies run between 30 and 50 percent, compared to 12 to 15 percent for large group, employer-sponsored insurance.[12])

In addition to driving Americans into less comprehensive health insurance policies and reducing their protection, analysts believe the McCain plan would have had little initial effect on the number of the uninsured.[13] However, within five years, the ranks of the uninsured would have expanded as the value of McCain's tax credit dropped relative to the increase in the price of insurance. And the cost of McCain's plan was also not inconsequential. It was estimated that the tax-related features of McCain's reform program would have run about $1.3 trillion over a ten year period, with the high-risk pools costing about

$70–$100 billion,[14] or even more.[15]) Interestingly, U.S. businesses, which are generally supportive of Republican economic initiatives, were unenthusiastic about the McCain plan.[16]

The scorecard for the McCain proposal read increased complexity, higher administrative and overhead costs, no restrictions on unnecessary care, no major reduction in the uninsured, and higher taxes for a number of Americans. It was not a reform program that even attempted to address all the aspects of the health care crisis.

## The Obama Health Care Plan

The Obama plan for health care reform relies on mandates to force businesses to buy health insurance for their employees or to pay a tax.[17] This is known as a "pay or play" option, with the tax collected helping to fund coverage for those without insurance. Some small businesses would be granted subsidies to help them insure their employees, and others would be exempt from the requirement. In addition, a new government health plan similar to Medicare would be created to allow individuals without insurance, and small businesses who wanted to obtain insurance for their employees, to purchase coverage at reasonable prices.[18] This National Health Plan (NHP) has also been described as being similar to one of the Federal Employees Health Benefits plans (FEHB) and costing in the same range.[19] (Some proponents have said it is like the plan utilized by members of Congress.)

There would also be another choice for coverage offered under the Obama plan. A national health insurance exchange or purchasing pool of private insurance would be available to uninsured individuals and small businesses. (This "insurance exchange" would be somewhat similar to the Massachusetts' Commonwealth Connector Authority, established under the state's reform plan in an attempt to provide affordable health insurance to those without coverage.) As a further step to allow access to everyone, medical underwriting on the basis of health status would be eliminated, with private insurers no longer able to deny coverage or charge higher premiums to people with preexisting conditions. Low-income individuals would also receive subsidies to help them purchase insurance. Though adults could still elect to go without insurance, all children would be required to have coverage. Those children whose families could not afford private insurance would be covered by an expansion of Medicaid or the State Children's Health Insurance Program.[20] Another measure in the Obama plan includes a federal reinsurance program to protect businesses against expenses related to worker's catastrophic medical events.

To help control costs, faster utilization of electronic medical records would be promoted. (Obama wants $50 billion to be invested in health information technology.[21]) There would also be a focus on disease management, preventive care and public health measures, paying providers for performance and outcomes, and cutting the extra payments to private Medicare plans—Medicare Advantage. While all of these objectives sound worthwhile, the actual cost savings that would be generated if they were implemented, or whether there even would be savings, is unsettled. (Three of Obama's economic advisors have said that Obama's reform proposals could have produced $214 billion in savings in 2009,[22] $77 billion of which would supposedly have come from the use of computerized health records, which clearly was unattainable.) Obama's reform plan also permits Medicare to negotiate prices with drug companies, which should result in definite savings. However, in terms of the total cost of health care, it would be relatively modest. Another feature of the Obama plan is his desire to use alternative methods for resolving medical malpractice suits, an example of which is the University of Michigan Health System model.[23] This involves investigating medical errors, admitting and apologizing for them when they have occurred, and compensating patients even if there hasn't been a lawsuit. Obama also mentions reducing medical costs by "removing incentives for unnecessary care."[24] Though this sounds like an important step, he does not articulate how he would get it done.

Those favoring Obama's health care reform program cite its utilization of both a private and public pathway to medical coverage as a positive aspect. Though they believe that administrative costs could be cut by reduced marketing and increased competition, there is no hard data to support that conviction. In fact, heightened competition might lead to more marketing in an attempt to attract enrollees. How Obama's plan would play out in terms of coverage is difficult to estimate. Whether businesses would pay the tax or insure their employees would depend on the economic circumstances. They would obviously weigh the cost of the tax versus the cost of offering insurance to their employees, and without knowing what the cost of either one would be, the results cannot be predicted.

Given the new range of options for health care coverage, many currently uninsured Americans would probably obtain coverage under the Obama plan. But there would not be universal access. Increased coverage for lower income Americans would be related to the subsidies that were provided, as well as the actual cost of the insurance. Though the cost might be lower than under the present system, it would still be substantial and it is likely that numerous individuals who are now uninsured would remain so under the Obama plan. (It is also possible that at some point in the future, individual mandates to purchase insurance could be introduced by Obama if universal or near universal coverage were not achieved.)

Analysts note that if the National Health Plan featured in the Obama program were to have similar cost and coverage to the most popular of the FEHB plans, it would not be affordable without major subsidies to moderate the premiums.[25] This raises concerns about the fiscal viability of the plan. Lowering the benefits would reduce the cost of the plan, but would shift more of the expenses of care to the enrollees, many of whom would be unable to pay. Subsidies would also be required for many of the private plans being offered through the national Health Insurance Exchange if benefits were at the same levels as the National Health Plan. The cost of such coverage might be unsustainable and make lower benefits a necessity. Whatever benefits were decided upon by the government would also apply to employer-based health insurance and the play-or-pay option.

Paying for the program Obama envisions is a matter of controversy. In addition to the payroll taxes that would be collected from businesses that did not insure their employees, its proponents estimate that $50 to $65 billion in new federal spending annually would be needed.[26] (Jonathan Gruber, a health economist at MIT puts this figure at $102 billion.[27]) Though the Obama plan anticipates raising these funds by allowing the Bush tax cuts for families making over $250,000 to expire, the Congressional Budget Office (CBO) has already incorporated the demise of these cuts into its projections after 2010. This means that additional revenues will not be available to meet congressional budget rules (assuming Obama's other areas of cost savings are not endorsed by the CBO), and substantial new revenues may have to be raised to implement the program. Obama's plan has not considered this possibility. He also claims that his proposal will save families $2,500 annually, an assertion that is not based on hard data.[28] Perhaps the greatest impediment to the Obama program is the amount of the federal subsidies that will be required to expand coverage—funding that will grow rapidly and will not be supportable either fiscally or politically.[29]

Though more Americans would obtain health care coverage under the Obama plan than under the plan McCain envisioned, both contain major flaws. These include the complexity of the programs, an unwillingness to address the issue of unnecessary care, uncertainty regarding the reduction of administrative expenses, and the large numbers of Americans who would probably continue to be uninsured. An article in *Health Affairs* in September 2008 that examined the Obama health care plan noted, "Since the government would bear the full liability for all health costs exceeding the affordability standard, there would be a strong incentive to continue the behavior that has caused health care spending to grow at alarming rates over the past decades."[30] One of the authors of this statement, Dr Joseph Antos, said in another recent analysis that the Obama plan, in "failing to address the perverse incentives that drive health care spending inexorably upward, making insurance unaffordable for millions and shaping (or misshaping) the practice of medicine, will leave us worse off than we are today."[31]

To summarize, the Obama plan does not realistically address the health care crisis at hand with a comprehensive program that provides universal access to care, along with significant savings. It is another attempt at incrementalism that will not work.

(There is also the issue of preventive care, which both reform plans claim will result in considerable cost savings—a concept that has been contested by some workers in the field. Dr. H. Gilbert Welch, a professor at the Dartmouth Institute for Health Policy and Clinical Practice at Dartmouth, noted in a recent article in the *New York Times* that "The myth is that like magic, preventive medicine will simultaneously reduce costs and improve health."[32] In actuality, it is possible that preventive medicine could increase costs, as prevention now means early diagnosis, as well as health promotion. This involves taking healthy people and subjecting them to various screening tests in attempts to spot problems at an early stage—an approach that costs money instead of saving money. The screening tests themselves are costly, and the follow-up tests and procedures may even be more expensive. Though some individuals may benefit by having a treatable illness found before it gets out of hand, very few of those screened fall into this category. And there are occasional adverse effects in those who are tested or treated. The risk/benefit ratio in this type of preventive care is unclear.)

With Obama as president and the Democrats in control of Congress, it is likely that major health care reform will be passed before the next federal elections, though its provisions are yet to be determined. Given the recent financial crisis and the government intervention that has occurred in the markets, it is possible that some type of comprehensive reform would have a chance for Congressional approval. This is contingent on legislators understanding the scope of the health care crisis and what it portends for the country in terms of immediate economic hardship and the future pain of unfunded liabilities. There must also be the realization that comprehensive reform does not have to require additional federal funding and can save money while providing universal access to care. The statistics supporting these claims are out there. The politicians just have to analyze them and come to the proper conclusions without ideological blinders.

## Other Plans for Health Care Reform

Though the McCain and Obama plans for health care reform have received the most attention, a number of other proposals have been advanced by various economists and politicians. These run the gamut in scope and form, including single-payer systems, health savings accounts, tax credits for health insurance, and increased competition between insurance companies in a free-market system. To increase access to health care for poor people, government subsidies for insurance is required by many of these programs. While some of them assert they will be able to lower administrative expenses, none of them address how to eliminate defensive medicine and the incentives physicians have to increase services that result in unnecessary care. No reform program can be successful without a solution to this problem.

The Massachusetts model for reform has been suggested as a possible alternative method for providing universal access to heath care, either on a federal or state-by-state basis.[33] The program was formulated on the concept of shared responsibility between citizens, businesses, and government, with everyone who does not have health insurance mandated to buy it. For those below a certain income level who were deemed unable to afford the coverage, subsidies were to be provided, with an insurance pool reducing premiums for small groups and individuals.[34] The insurance pool, or what has been called the "Massachusetts Connector," was established to help people obtain coverage at reasonable prices, even if they had preexisting conditions. In addition to premium payments from individuals buying insurance, funding of the program comes from the state and federal governments, plus assessments on hospitals, insurers, and employers. Businesses that do not offer health insurance to their employees must pay a fee, with individuals also penalized with an assessment if they don't obtain coverage. It is hoped that this penalty will help bring young, healthy people into the program and lower costs by spreading the risk of illness around.

In the two years it has been in existence, the Massachusetts program has been successful in reducing the percentage of the uninsured in the state, which is now the lowest in the country.[35] However, over one-third of those who were uninsured initially still remain so, many of them unable to afford the premiums. Even more discouraging, perhaps, is the fact that the costs of the program have escalated more than was predicted, with greater subsidies required, and no constraints on unnecessary care or administrative expenditures. And the plan is inordinately complex. Undercutting the positive aspects of the program has been the lack of primary care physicians in the state to handle the surge of recent enrollees.[36] The question remains whether the state will be able to somehow control spending for health care under this program, or whether the growth in expenditures will simply be unsustainable.

The Massachusetts plan initially engendered enthusiasm for similar programs in other states, but that has subsequently evaporated as its cost became more evident. A California bill structured on the Massachusetts' strategy was rejected in January 2008 by a state senate committee, despite the backing of Governor Schwarzenegger, because of the pessimistic cost projections it produced.[37] It does not appear that a Massachusetts-type plan is ready for primetime as the basis for federal health care reform.

Florida passed a bill in May 2008 with the hope that it would reduce the percentage of those lacking health insurance in the state, which is the fourth highest in the nation at 21 percent.[38] The legislation allowed insurers to issue stripped-down policies that did not cover many services, which could then be sold inexpensively to those unable to afford more inclusive policies. Governor Charlie Crist of Florida lauded these new options, noting that they would cost the state nothing. However, similar insurance coverage that has previously been tried elsewhere has not been very successful. Consumers have been reluctant to purchase this insurance knowing that they would still be left with unaffordably high out-of-pocket costs if they subsequently required care. This type of plan does not reduce overall health care spending, and it would not significantly increase access to care.

Tom Price, a Republican congressman from Georgia who is an orthopedic surgeon, has introduced a reform plan that would give individuals the opportunity to purchase health insurance with pretax dollars, as is the case for those who obtain coverage from their employers.[39] His program would also offer tax deductions and credits to those who cannot afford the premiums. The cost of this proposal has not been determined, but it would certainly be quite expensive. Again, there are no provisions to limit incentives for physicians to generate unnecessary care, nor to reduce administrative expenditures.

The Mayo Clinic has produced a plan for universal coverage that was created by a panel of experts on health care.[40] This proposal has private insurance companies mandated to offer people standard plans with various choices, similar to the Federal Employees Health Benefits Plan. Under this program, there could be no rejections of anyone who wanted coverage, even those with preexisting conditions. Individuals would purchase these policies, with employers' assistance in some cases, with those unable to afford the premiums receiving government subsidies to help them. There would be portability of the policies as well, allowing workers the freedom to change jobs. While this plan addresses the problem of universal coverage, it offers no realistic suggestions to constrain costs.

In the past, the American Medical Association has mainly played a reactive role in opposition to health care reform. However, with the knowledge that some sort of reform bill is likely to pass in the next Congress, it has proposed its own plan in an attempt to influence the debate. Endorsing the idea of universal health coverage, AMA board member Joseph Annis stated, "Everyone should have health insurance. Be able to choose it. Take it state to state."[41] The AMA concept is to provide coverage for the uninsured by establishing a voucher or tax credit program, with financial incentives to the insurance companies to accept at-risk patients with pre-existing conditions. The AMA plan was created in collaboration with 15 other national organizations involved in health care and calls itself the Health Care Coverage Coalition for the Uninsured. Among its members are the American Hospital Association, America's Health Insurance Plans (an association of health insurance companies), and the American Association of Retired Persons (AARP). The three major facets of the plan are:

Enable uninsured individuals and families to purchase coverage of their own choosing.

Make subsidies available—via tax credits or vouchers—to those who cannot otherwise obtain health insurance.

Foster market reforms that encourage the creation of innovative and affordable health insurance options.[42]

It must be remembered that there are obvious conflicts of interest involving the organizations that devised the plan and what they are suggesting. Indeed, there are a number of problems with the AMA proposal that make it a nonstarter in terms of a viable solution to the health care crisis. One of the AMA's main goals has been the preservation of physicians' income and the goal of the insurance companies has been to maintain their status in the health care industry. Thus, in the proposal there are no constraints placed on the incentives that drive physicians to provide unnecessary care (and enhance their remuneration). In addition, under the AMA plan, private insurance companies with their administrative bureaucracies and high overhead are projected to continue in charge of health care management, an arrangement that has been responsible for many of the current problems. The AMA program is also inordinately complex and fails to specify how it will pay for the government subsidies it envisions and for the expenditures from the influx of new patients that will flood the system.

Since private insurance companies, with their obligations to shareholders (and executives) to maximize profit, will still be running health care, co-pays and deductibles for coverage will remain high, and care will continue to be unaffordable for many patients. Some, in fact, will probably be unable to pay for basic insurance even with the subsidies granted by the government. One can also expect the pattern of denials for care and rejections of payment by the insurance companies to continue whenever it is feasible to do so. There are some similarities in the AMA proposal and the McCain reform plan, and both flounder for many of the same reasons. The inability to rein in costs is undoubtedly the most important.

Though Obama's vision for health care reform has been in the public domain for some time, he has left it to the Senate and House committees to shape the reform legislation, rather than trying to impose his plan on them. A number of long time legislative stalwarts, among them Senators Ted Kennedy and Max Baucus, have their own ideas about health care reform and it is uncertain what shape the program will ultimately take. It is clear however, that none of the designers wish to challenge the major stakeholders in the current system (i.e., the insurance industry, organized medicine, the pharmaceutical industry, and the trial lawyers). Unfortunately, this means it is likely that market-based solutions will continue to play a large role in whatever plan is crafted, and that simplicity and sound cost-constraints will not be included.

## The Health Care Systems of Other Nations

Every industrialized nation, aside from the United States, provides universal health care for its citizens, though there are differences in how this is accomplished. As the United States moves in the direction of universal access, there are some lessons that can be learned from these other systems, both in terms of what works well and what does not. With that said, given its history of past failures and the strong opposition that is bound to arise from entrenched interests, the United States must find its own unique path towards that still elusive goal of health care coverage for all (with realistic cost constraints). Capsule summaries of some other nations' health care systems follow.

### United Kingdom

The English health care system, known as the National Health Service (NHS), was established in England and Wales in 1946 through an act of Parliament and a year later in Scotland. The system is administered separately in the four parts of the United Kingdom, which has a population of about 60 million. The mission of the NHS is to provide free health care services for everyone, financed by general taxes. Since its inception, the program has evolved considerably, driven by changes in medical care, the cost of services, and the expensive new technology that has been developed over the years. There are various layers in the system of administrative and executive functions, with a number of redundancies and overlapping roles that affect responsibility for providing care. The person in charge is the secretary of state for Health who decides on the allocation of funds and is accountable to Parliament for the performance of the NHS. Below the secretary is the Department of Health and the NHS Executive, the generator of strategic planning for the entire system.[43],[44] Below the Department of Health are 28 Strategic Health Authorities (SHAs) that shape health care for the regions they cover and integrate the national priorities for care.

Under the SHAs, primary and secondary "trusts" have been established to deliver care. There are 303 Primary Care Trusts (PCTs) throughout England that interact with patients and provide services through general practitioners, dentists, pharmacists, opticians, district nursing, and community health services. (GPs and dentists are paid for each of their registered patients, but are also permitted to see private patients. A new pay-for-performance program was also instituted for GPs in 2004, with $3.2 billion allotted,[45] but was apparently unsuccessful.) The care is rendered locally in the area where the covered population lives, in doctors' offices, in community health centers, and even in people's homes. Seventy-five percent of the NHS budget is allocated for the PCTs to fund patient care.[46] There are lay boards to provide oversight of the PCTs and professional committees to counsel the boards and the PCTs about clinical matters. Various other PCT committees play different roles. The GPs act as gatekeepers, directing patients to specialists when needed for more complex diagnostic testing and therapy.

In addition to providing primary care services, the PCTs "are responsible for buying almost all of the health care, both primary and secondary, required by the populations they serve."[47] Using the funds they receive from the Department of Health, they must decide what they will spend on various services for the people in their local area. The PCTs commission health care from the GPs, hospitals, and other providers, paying them an agreed fee, or on a contractual basis.[48] If the PCTs go over budget because of unforeseen circumstances, or because too much was allotted for a particular service or item, they may be forced to cut back on other services or to ask the Department of Health for more funds, which may not be forthcoming. The high cost of certain drugs, particularly the newer ones for cancer therapy, can decimate the budgets of the PCTs and lead to disputes over approvals. To meet their budgets, staffs may be laid off, new technology deferred, and old equipment overbooked. If the PCTs fail to meet their financial goals by the end of the fiscal year, their boards of directors can be dismissed.

The NHS Trusts for secondary health care encompasses hospitals, specialty care, ambulances, mental health services, and learning disability services. Two-hundred ninety organizations run the hospitals and treatment centers and provide specialty care in about 1,600 NHS hospitals.[49] The NHS of Great Britain is one of the world's largest employers; as of March 2005 it had 1.3 million employees.[50] (Unlike the GPs who receive a capitated fee for each registered patient, the professionals responsible for hospital and specialty services are paid a salary.) With costs continuously rising, the NHS has been under financial pressure for some time, and has been looking for ways, to save money. (In fact, some trusts have been running deficits.) As of April 2007, patients were being charged £6.88 (pounds) per prescription, regardless of the cost of the medication. However, this fee was waived for those over 60 or under 16, as well as for people with low incomes or certain illnesses. There were also charges for dental work, which were quite reasonable by U.S. standards. (Though dentists do subcontracted work from the NHS, they have separate private practices as well, with many of them gravitating in that direction.) In the last ten years, there has been more outsourcing of medical services to the private sector, when spare capacity exists, to try and obtain faster evaluation and treatment for patients. As a result, more private hospitals are being built by groups of investors who see an opportunity for profit.

Though many patients are satisfied and appreciative of the National Health Service, significant problems exist. With its free services for everyone, demand has grown inordinately, as the costs of care have been invisible to patients. To try and control expenditures, the NHS has given physicians rules, which spell out what may and may not be done. These require doctors to deny services to their patients, which can be stressful for both parties. With limited resources, there are also long waits for some services, particularly, consultations with specialists, high-tech tests, and complex treatments. (As an example, there has been a dearth of facilities to handle all the patients needing renal dialysis.) And some treatments are not covered by the NHS because they are not deemed cost-effective, even though they may provide benefits for some patients. For the above reasons, some of the more affluent citizens have opted for private care and paying twice for services—once through their taxes that go to the NHS and then directly to the private physicians for the services.

Another dilemma not anticipated at the time the NHS was started is how to deal with patients who have complex illnesses and want to pay privately for some of their therapy, while getting the rest free from the NHS.[51] This is particularly an issue with some of the new biopharmaceutical cancer treatments that can cost tens to hundreds of thousands of dollars and are not covered by the NHS. Patients who pay privately for these treatments become responsible for all the costs of care, as allowing special treatments or upgrades in care for those who can pay more goes against the founding principles of the NHS. This problem is exacerbated by the inequities found throughout the health service, with some drugs being available in some regions but not in others. Great variation also exists in how much is spent per capita on cancer care in different parts of the country. There are political pressures as well that buffet the system, with requests to increase overall or targeted spending, and to provide different kinds of treatment for patients. Whatever the criticisms of the NHS may be,

supporters point to the fact that the health outcomes in England are comparable to those in other countries and at lower cost.

## Canada

Canada has a large land mass with a population of only 33 million. The
Canada Health Act passed in 1984 entitled all legal residents of Canada to obtain
medically necessary care from practitioners as outpatients, or in hospitals,
through universal insurance without co-pays.[52] (The health care system in
Canada is known unofficially as medicare, lowercase.) In reality, there is not a
single Canadian health care system, but a number of provincial systems with
each province administering its own insurance program with its own identifica-
tion cards. Though all the plans must cover the services delineated in the
Canada Health Act, there is variation in what other services each province will
pay for and how much will be paid. Included in the variable category are prescription drug coverage, mental health, dental services, vision care, and long
term care. Additional coverage may be offered in some provinces for seniors or
children, those with conditions such as cancer or AIDS, and low income families. Generally, uncovered services are paid for out-of-pocket or by private insurance. But whatever care is deemed medically necessary must be picked up by the
government. (The site of care and whether it should be in-patient or out-patient
may also determine whether services are covered.) About 70 percent of the
country's health care spending is of public origin, with the remainder being paid
through insurance or directly from patients. Aside from general tax revenues,
with the federal government disbursing money to the provincial authorities,
each province raises additional funds in different ways. These include modest
health care premiums and employer health care taxes. One of the positive
aspects of the medicare system in Canada is its low overhead and administrative
costs, with the provincial plans in Canada running about 1 percent.[53] (This com-
pares to 15–25 percent or more in the United States.)

The delivery of health care is in the hands of both private and public providers,
who are paid by the provinces for the services they render. Almost all physicians
are self-employed, as members of groups or solo practitioners, and work on a fee-
for-service basis. Specialists and hospital-based physicians are paid fee-for-service
by the provincial health authorities. Recently, there have been some attempts to
employ alternative payment methods, including capitation, episode-based remuneration, and mixed models. Physicians' fees are fixed by the provincial governments, with periodic increases resulting from negotiations with the provincial
medical associations. This establishes a pool from which physicians can be paid at
an agreed-upon schedule. If this pool exceeds its budget, there is a "claw back"
clause in most agreements, under which physician payments can be reduced to
eliminate the excess. This can lead to conflicts among primary care physicians and
specialists about how the funding pool should be allotted.

Canadian hospitals are generally nonprofit and associated with religious or
charitable groups. However, in some provinces these institutions have been joined

together in quasiprivate bodies known as regional health authorities that are usually controlled by the provincial governments. Investments in expensive new technology, such as imaging machines, are frequently not forthcoming from the authorities. This has resulted in patients in some locales having long waits to obtain necessary diagnostic testing, which can delay treatment and affect prognoses. Patients may face considerable delays for elective operations, such as joint replacements and cataract extraction. A shortage of primary care physicians has also occurred in some areas, making it more difficult for patients to obtain acute care. Laboratory services are generally provided by for-profit corporations.

Provincial governments may or may not allow private clinics to operate, but private care is utilized by only a small percentage of the Canadian population. Private surgical procedures are limited by the overhead associated with running a private surgical center, which is difficult to cover given the allowable fees. Policies regarding private surgical services vary from province to province, and quality assurance and oversight may not always be up to par. (Public funding can not be utilized in private facilities as it would go against certain concepts inherent in the Canada Health Act.) Nevertheless, there are functioning private hospitals, and Quebec permits its residents to buy private insurance.

Criticism of the Canadian health care system revolves around inadequate investment in new technology, hospital and medical center infrastructures, and the long waits for certain tests and procedures. There is also a shortage of physicians, both PCPs and specialists. This can at least be partially explained by a brain drain of physicians (and nurses) to the United States, where they are able to earn more money and may have better working conditions. The fact that each province handles health care and services somewhat differently fragments the system and adds a degree of complexity.

### Germany

The Federal Republic of Germany has sixteen states with a population of 85 million people. State-regulated plans provide most Germans with their health insurance, with funding coming from several sources. Having coverage is mandatory, but various options are available. Those who work contribute 13.99 percent of the nonexempt portion of their income towards their insurance, with half paid by the employee and half paid by the employer.[54] Low-income workers pay a lower percentage of their wages as a contribution, averaging about 4 percent, with subsidies for the poor and the unemployed. Long-term care insurance is also required for which Germans contribute 1.7 percent of their income.[55] After retirement at age 65, people no longer have to pay into the programs, but they continue to receive coverage.[56] Those who are self-employed do not participate in the state plan and are obligated to get private insurance. Interestingly, public sector employees are not covered by the state plan and must also get private insurance, though they receive reimbursement for a portion of their health care costs. High income earners are allowed to drop out of the state-regulated plans and obtain private insurance if they wish. There are 7 million Germans who have private health insurance.[57] Health care coverage under this system is virtually universal, with less than 0.2 percent of Germans lacking coverage.[58] Because of rising costs, additional charges for the state plan were instituted in 2004.[59] These included €10 (Euros) per quarter to visit a general practitioner and contributions towards the costs of drugs, wound dressings, rehabilitation treatment, inpatient hospital care (€9 per day), and so forth.

Physicians' fees, hospital costs, chronic care, and some dental care are covered by both private and state regulated insurance plans. Physicians and hospitals deal directly with the insurance carriers for any care provided, including diagnostic tests, treatment, and drugs. General practitioners work on a fee-for-service basis, with the fees negotiated with the state plan.[60] Private patients may be charged higher fees by physicians, but it is up to the insurance company to decide whether the charge is reasonable and whether to pay it. The government has negotiated discounts on medications with the drug companies to try and keep costs in check. Patients can use any approved primary care physician or specialist. Those who have the state regulated plans and those with private plans utilize the same hospitals and receive the same care, though some hospitals have designated particular wards for private patients.

Physicians work either in private practice or hospital settings. Private practitioners, who can be PCPs or specialists, are self-employed and have their own offices. When problems arise that require hospitalization, patients are referred to the hospital doctors. Physicians who are hospital-based are employed by those institutions. Some surgeons are permitted to have reserved beds in the hospitals where they operate. Though there have been major waiting times for surgery, consultations, and procedures in the past, this appears to have improved in recent years.

Because physicians are paid on the basis of the services they provide patients, there have been a number of cases of billing fraud, where doctors charged insurance companies for procedures or treatments that were never performed.[61] In addition to fraud, because of the financial incentives, it is likely that there is a large amount of unnecessary care in the German system. This was confirmed by the German Health Ministry in May 2003 when the prevalence of "superfluous, insufficient or inappropriate care" was decried.[62] Malpractice has apparently been on the increase. Other problems with the German system include meager screening facilities for breast cancer and a lack of attention to palliative care. There is poor coordination as well between the hospitals and outpatient providers, and limited support from social services.

### France

France has a population of about 62 million. The World Health Organization recently described French health care as the best in the world, ranking the United States as 37th.[63] Supporting this disparity in standing, the average life expectancy in France was found to be two years longer than in the United States, with infant mortality nearly half that of the United States. In addition, deaths from chronic illnesses, such as diabetes, heart disease, and pulmonary disease, were considerably lower than in the United States. Yet, even though their outcomes are better, the French spend much less per capita on health care than in the United States—$3,500 per person versus $6,100 in the United States (figures for April 2008.[64] which equates to 10.7 percent of France's GDP, vs. 16 percent of the U.S. GDP[65]). Why is the French health care system producing better results at a lower cost?

The French have universal health care, which is sustained by a blend of public and private financing.[66] The public health insurance system (PHIS) was established in 1945 and augmented over the years to cover all legal residents.[67] The main fund encompasses 80 percent of the population, with two other funds that insure agricultural workers and the self-employed. Employer and employee contributions underwrite the funds along with personal income taxes. However, as costs have escalated, income taxes have been employed for an increasing percentage of the financing. The insurance funds are basically private aggregations run jointly by union federations and business federations under government supervision.[68] Because of the diffusion of responsibility and management, there has been conflict at times among the different parties over policies and objectives. While parliament may allocate a certain amount of public funding to the health care system, the cabinet fixes reimbursement rates and decides how much public money will actually be distributed to the insurance funds. Then the funds negotiate with medical unions to set the fees for services, trying to keep spending at a break even point. The final results however, may lead to acrimony and not satisfy all the involved parties.

The French government is responsible for planning for the health care system. The State decides on the requirements for hospital beds: how many are needed and where they should be located. There are both public and private for-profit hospitals, roughly divided in a ratio of two-thirds to one-third. Training and teaching occurs at the public hospitals, whose wards provide most of the in-patient care. The private hospitals are more surgically oriented and are generally paid on a fee-for-service basis, but episode-based compensation will eventually be the norm at both private and public institutions. The State also determines the need for medical technology, such as CT machines, MRI, and PET scanners, and their placement, as well as operating rooms, emergency rooms, ICUs, and so forth. Specialized services, such as transplant teams, dialysis facilities, and radiation treatment centers, are also allocated by the health authorities who have responsibility for quality and safety issues as well.

About three-quarters of health expenditures are covered by public health insurance. Of the remainder, half is paid out-of-pocket and half is covered by supplementary private policies.[69] This supplemental insurance is taken out by about 85 percent of the population, either individually or through groups. Because of a steady increase in health care spending and consumption, copayments were instituted to try and keep costs under control. But these copayments have grown larger over time, particularly for ambulatory care. (There are no deductibles.) Of the fixed tariff (fee) to visit a physician, the patient is now responsible for 30 percent.[70] In addition, about one-sixth of primary care physicians and two-fifths of specialists are permitted to charge more than the established fees. As poor citizens are unable to afford the co-pays and don't have private supplementary insurance, a public insurance program was enacted in 2000 to guarantee the poor full access to care. Providers are not allowed to charge these patients anything above the established fees. In spite of the problems with funding, because of negotiations with the union federations, a number of questionable services are covered by the public insurance fund, such as "treatments" in thermal spas. But when patients have serious afflictions such as cancer, severe coronary artery disease, or diabetes, medical care is reimbursed completely. Even expensive cancer drugs are fully covered and hospital charges are regulated by the government.

There are many more physicians and hospital beds per capita in France than in the United States, and patients are able to select their own doctors and have access to any specialist. Though referrals to specialists were not required in the past and there was no gatekeeping, this is in the process of changing. The system was perhaps too patient friendly, allowing them to visit as many physicians (including specialists) as often as they liked. Now, however, patients must register with a PCP before seeing a specialist, or they will have less of the fee covered by their insurance.

Physicians earn only about a third of the income of their peers in the United States, about $55,000 per year.[71] On the other hand, medical school is fully subsidized by the state, so there are no educational loans that have to be paid back. As another benefit for physicians, the government pays two-thirds of their social security tax, an amount that is generally about 40 percent of income. Physicians may also earn more by increasing their patient volume or by generating additional services and procedures (the same strategy that is responsible for raising health care costs in the United States). And specialists who have been in a hospital practice for at least four years are able to set their own fees, though social pressures have generally kept these charges under control. (Some physicians choose to work outside the insurance system and charge patients whatever they believe will be accepted.) Another helpful factor for physicians is that malpractice premiums are minuscule by U.S. standards. (Twenty-five percent of French physicians are employed by public hospitals, 11 percent in other public facilities, and 56 percent in private practices.[72] Half of all physicians are specialists.)

As with all national health care systems, the French have some problems with theirs. French health care is expensive (though considerably less so than U.S. health care), and to fund it, employees have to pay about 21 percent of their income for the national health system, half of which is contributed by their employers.[73] (Though Americans pay much less in taxes, the total cost of health care for most individuals is much higher, factoring in the expenses of insurance, co-pays, and deductibles, as well as out-of-pocket spending on drugs and services that are not covered.) France also has to deal with rising health care expenditures and is running an annual deficit in this area. Given the universal access to primary care physicians and specialists, along with expensive tests and treatments, with costs for the most part invisible to patients, constraining spending is proving to be difficult. Though physician incomes are not adequate to consistently attract the highest caliber of student, the financial incentives that physicians have to increase services and procedures continue to drive up costs. There are also questions about cost/effectiveness and efficiency in the way certain aspects of care are managed, which need to be resolved. But in spite of the flaws that may exist, the French health care system generally provides all of its citizens with a high caliber of care.

### Japan

Japan is a heavily industrialized country of 127 million people sustained by an export-oriented economy. Though its citizens have the longest life expectancy of any nation, it spends about half the amount per capita on health care as the United States.[74] While diet and life style play an important role in the health and survival of its population, its universal health care system is an important factor. All Japanese are mandated to have health insurance, acquiring it through work or via community-based insurers. Employees of medium-to-large companies, national or local governments, private schools, and small businesses are all covered by Employee Health Insurance.[75] The premiums are determined by salary, with half being paid by the employer and half by the employee. About 4 percent of each person's salary goes for this insurance. There is a 20 percent co-pay for hospitalization and 30 percent for out-patient care, with a copayment as well for medications. When a certain point is reached, however, the insurance pays all costs. The unemployed, including retirees and students, agricultural, forestry or fishery workers, and those who are self-employed are covered by National Health Insurance. Premiums and copayments are similar to those for Employee Health Insurance. People over 70 are covered by a national health program for the elderly, with funding from the two main plans. Insurers must provide coverage for everyone and are not allowed to deny claims. They are also not permitted to make a profit, with excess funds carried over to the following year. The government pays the premium for those who are poor.

Physicians are in private practice and own about 80 percent of the hospitals, with the remaining 20 percent being state-owned teaching hospitals.[76] By law, however, all hospitals must be nonprofit in their operations. Hospital-based physicians are paid by salary and private physicians on a fee-for-service basis. Private physicians are not given hospital privileges, but must see patients in their offices or in clinics. Hospitals also provide outpatient services. The Japanese visit physicians about three times as frequently as Americans and have access to any specialist. There are also no waiting lists to consult doctors or have procedures. Hospital stays last longer than in the United States, and there are about twice as many scans (MRIs, CTs, etc.) done per capita compared to the United States. The reason these scans and other services are so affordable in

Japan is because prices and fees are set by the government. Every two years there are negotiations between the Health Ministry and various health industry players that establishes the price for all services, procedures, medications, and other treatments. Physicians and other providers are required to abide by this price schedule. With universal access and low cost, every person is able to obtain care for any medical problem, and no one is bankrupted due to medical expenses.

The downside to this system is that physicians are paid very poorly for their services and many have to find other ways to supplement their incomes. Some doctors sell nonprescription drugs or equipment to their patients, have vending machines for food and drinks in their offices, and charge for parking.[77] There is also no differentiation between general practitioners and specialists in terms of fees, with both receiving the same fee for each service.[78] Because of this, most physicians in private practice tend to manage all of their patients' problems across the board. In addition, prescribing and dispensing medications is not legally separated in Japan, which can cause conflicts of interest with the over-prescribing of drugs, along with kickbacks from drug companies.[79] About half the hospitals are in financial trouble because of the low level of reimbursement. The number of scans and the long duration of hospitalizations make Japanese care less cost-effective as well. Perhaps the most critical challenge to the Japanese health system, however, is demographic. With an aging population and a shrinking workforce, it will be difficult for employers and workers to support health care for the growing number of retirees. The Ministry of Health has suggested the need for a radical overhaul of the health insurance system to cut down on accelerating costs, while still providing quality care.[80]

There is no common template for a health care system that is used by every nation. Each developed nation has created its own program to deliver health care to its people, which is different from every other, but commensurate with its culture and mores. However, there are certain characteristics of all these programs that are important for Americans to keep in mind. In every one, there is universal access to care and the process is less expensive than health care in the United States. (Health care in most nations is considered a basic human right.) From the dysfunctionality of the current U.S. system, a new program must be created that will provide universal coverage in a cost-effective manner.

## CHAPTER 8

# OBSTACLES TO COMPREHENSIVE REFORM

A good government implies two things: first, fidelity to the object of government, which is the happiness of the people; secondly, a knowledge of the means by which that object can be best attained.

—James Madison, *The Federalist Papers*[1]

The public and the political establishment may be considered as obstacles on the road to reform and must be sold on the need for comprehensive reform in order for it to become the law of the land. However, the program's most implacable and hostile opponents will be the lobbyists and the entrenched special interests they represent, who stand to lose money and power if the old system is dismantled and replaced. Included among the special interests are the American Medical Association (AMA) and organized medicine, the health insurance industry, the pharmaceutical and medical device industries, hospital organizations, and trial lawyers, all of whom will mobilize their resources to block the passage of comprehensive reform.

## The Public

Many Americans are relatively satisfied with their health care coverage (aside from cost) and may be neutral or ambivalent about the idea of comprehensive reform (though a certain percentage will embrace the concept). But before a comprehensive program can be enacted, a majority has to be convinced that the current system is floundering dangerously and needs to be thoroughly overhauled. Since the plans for reform thus far circulated have suggested only incremental changes, Americans have not been attuned to the idea of comprehensive reform with its far-reaching transformation and may be surprised, and perhaps frightened, by a proposal that recommends major changes. Along with most politicians, U.S. citizens are generally reluctant to alter the status quo. They need unassailable arguments laid out for them showing why change is necessary, with repeated reinforcement. Providing health care coverage to those who are uninsured may not be enough of a reason for a preponderance of Americans to back comprehensive reform. They must be made to understand the magnitude of the unfunded liabilities that are growing every day because of the costs of Medicare and Medicaid and of the risks to the economy of unfettered health care spending.

It is likely that the battle for health care reform will be largely fought in the court of public opinion, with the media used to influence Americans (and Congress) to oppose any major changes in the present system. The "Harry and Louise" campaign of the 1990s that savaged the Clinton health care proposals (which would not have worked anyway), will seem tame compared to the barrage of negative advertising that can be expected from the consortium of special interests. And of course, the old bogeyman of "socialized medicine" will be resurrected and featured prominently in attempts to frighten people about comprehensive reform. The task of counteracting the attack ads and of educating the public about the critical need for reform will fall to the advocates of change, including various foundations, policy institutes, academics, the politicians who are aware of the stakes and favor comprehensive reform, and those believers within the health care industry itself. But unless the polls show that the electorate is supportive of the changes being considered, it is unlikely that a critical mass of politicians will be bold enough to enact the necessary legislation. The changes are far too sweeping, with an effect on the economy and on every American's life, for politicians to be willing to step ahead of the crowd. The U.S. public must back comprehensive reform before Congress will pass the enabling measures.

## The Politicians and the Political Parties

The politicians who will oppose comprehensive reform if and when it is proposed as legislation fall into two categories. The first are the free-market ideologues wedded to the market as a panacea for all U.S. problems. These men and women are innately hostile to any governmental or quasigovernmental entity being given increased control over a section of the economy. The second are those politicians who are resistant to changes of any sort because they can't predict what the ramifications of those changes will be and would be hesitant to consider a dramatic reconfiguration of an industry responsible for 16 percent of the economy.

The free-marketeers will pose more of a problem to enacting comprehensive reform because their ideology is usually deep-seated, and they are less likely to consider nonmarket solutions to problems. They are generally against expanding government roles in any area and decry social assistance programs. Many of them also don't see health care reform as a priority, and the idea of a huge quasigovernmental centralized entity such as Universal Medicare managing U.S. health care would be an anathema to them. The free-marketeers are also antitax to the core and would be most reluctant to agree to any new tax/fee on businesses, even though it would be coming from money the businesses saved on their employees' health insurance under the new program. The most strongly committed of this group are right-wing Republicans who could conceivably block reform through a filibuster in the Senate, although the Democrats have a majority in both Houses. Sixty votes would be required in the Senate to invoke cloture and end the filibuster, allowing a bill on comprehensive reform to come to a vote. (It is more likely that a filibuster of health care reform could be overcome since Senator Arlen Specter of Pennsylvania switched from the Republican to the Democratic side of the aisle in April of 2009.)

However, as previously mentioned, some of these free-marketeers supported government bailouts of the banks in the 1980s and 1990s, along with the recent assistance and guarantees to distressed U.S. financial firms. Even though the bailouts clashed with their ideology, the measures were seen as imperative for the health of the economy and these free-market legislators acted responsibly. The continuing agricultural subsidies to farmers that many of these politicians promote out of political necessity are also contrary to their free-market ideology. And they cannot be blind to the disasters of the airline and electric utility deregulations that were done in the name of the market. As further evidence against market solutions to health care problems there is the disconcerting fact that private Medicare plans (Medicare Advantage) are more expensive to run than regular Medicare and require government subsidies to function. Perhaps all of these particulars will make the free-marketeers more amenable to the possibility of a nonmarket strategy to resolve the health care crisis, if they can be made to see that market forces do not work adequately where health care is concerned. But it is not likely that their ideology can be overcome.

More moderate Republicans and some Democrats might also be reluctant to back comprehensive reform because of a relative allegiance to the market, or simply because they have misgivings about legislating sweeping changes in an important sector of the economy. Elected officials often tend to follow the paths of least resistance, and many are naturally inclined to oppose change. But the views of these senators and representatives might not be as ingrained as those of the free-marketeers, and it may be easier to persuade them that far-reaching measures to bring health care spending under control are needed. Those who worry that Universal Medicare would just be another government program that drives up the national debt or requires new taxes could be shown the ways the program can actually save money, reduce unfunded liabilities, and shore up the economy. It would be up to the pragmatists to convince these legislators of the positive effects Universal Medicare will have and how important it is for the nation to have this reform bill passed.

Another concern for politicians in regard to the reform program would be the job losses that could result at a time when the economy is already weak and unemployment is high, which might upset some of their politically active constituents. This concern is realistic, but it still does not make sense to maintain extraneous jobs in a health care system that is dysfunctional and wastes huge sums of money. The cost savings alone should cancel out the argument about job losses.

Of course, those senators, congressmen, and congresswomen who favor comprehensive reform will have to deal with the multitude of lobbyists and special interests who will be opposed. Independent of party affiliation, politicians are in thrall to the lobbyists and special interests who are the source of much of their campaign funds, providing direct contributions, bundling, and sponsoring of fundraisers. Congress has not stood up to them during past confrontations involving health care, as evidenced by the Medicare drug bill, the recent controversy over Medicare's spending on medical equipment, and Congress's overturning Medicare cuts in physicians' reimbursement.[2,3] Officials who anger the special interests find them threatening to withdraw financial and other support and possibly back political adversaries. Even most liberal Democrats are willing to suspend their ideology and beliefs, rather than buck the more powerful special interests. Since the organizations that would be against comprehensive reform are among the most prolific contributors to political campaigns in Washington and maintain an army of lobbyists, it will take particular courage for lawmakers to support comprehensive reform legislation and face their wrath.

Having a Democrat in the White House and a Democratic majority in both houses of Congress means that comprehensive reform might at least get a hearing. Though Obama's reform plan does not even approach the level of change in the health care system that is necessary, there are some Democrats who have favored a single-payer system as part of reform. The Democrats also seem to be more pragmatic in entertaining possible solutions to the health care crisis, and it was the Democrats under Lyndon Johnson who were able to pass the original Medicare program. There are two suppositions that the president and legislators must accept if they are to promote comprehensive reform. The first is that health care spending is jeopardizing the long term soundness of the U.S. economy. The second is that comprehensive reform can staunch the bleeding and bring runaway health care costs under control, unlike the partial measures that have been proposed. They may not initially like the medicine that is being prescribed, but they will realize that it must be swallowed if the patient is to be returned to good health.

## The Lobbyists

The lobbyists are men and women whose allegiance and marketing skills are for sale to the highest bidder. Some, however, tend to work exclusively for conservative causes, while others have a liberal outlook. Not withstanding their political stances, they have been hired by organized medicine, the pharmaceutical and medical device industries, the hospital industry, and the trial lawyers to try and block passage of any threatening components of health care reform. They have been successful in the past in thwarting reform legislation and will use whatever means is available to them to meet that goal again. Included will be attack ads in all the media, and the use of so-called experts and talking heads on television and the radio. These pundits will provide dire warnings about how comprehensive reform will destroy U.S. medicine by lowering quality and not allowing doctors to practice the way they want. As mentioned, the lobbyists will also try to intimidate and cajole House members and Senators to reject reform, raising the possibility of increased campaign funding for them if they are cooperative, or support for political opponents if they are not. (The health care sector is among the largest contributors to the campaigns of presidential, senatorial, and congressional candidates on both sides of the aisle.[4])

## The Special Interests

### Organized Medicine

Organized medicine's most unyielding champion has been the AMA, which has opposed virtually every proposal for health care reform throughout the twentieth century, including Medicare. Whenever national reform appeared to be on the horizon, the AMA raised its voice to resist the movement, using the specter of socialized medicine repeatedly as a scare tactic. Aside from the passage of Medicare and Medicaid in 1965, the AMA has been successful in all of its efforts to block reform, hiring additional lobbyists, and generating more funds from its members whenever a battle was imminent. There is no question that the AMA would again play a major role in attempting to subvert any health care reform legislation that included significant cost constraints, as these are likely to reduce many physicians' incomes. Indeed, since the collapse of the Clintons' attempt at reform in the 1990s, which the AMA also fought against, the organization's main activity has been as an advocate for higher reimbursement for physicians, challenging Medicare and the insurance companies. But today's AMA is not as strong as it has been in the past. Fewer than one-third of U.S. physicians can now be counted as paying members, and it no longer speaks for all of medicine.

However, the AMA is only one of a number of medical organizations that would take up the cudgel against comprehensive reform. The various professional associations representing surgical and medical specialists can be expected to join the battle, going all out to prevent enactment of reform measures that might negatively affect their members' incomes. These trade groups will find the ideas of placing physicians on salary, or reducing the disparity between procedure-oriented specialists and primary care practitioners, particularly repugnant, and they will aggressively work to defeat them. Of course, it is the specialist members of these organizations who are making the most money currently, given the way reimbursement is structured. Many of them who generate the largest incomes are also responsible for much of the unnecessary care patients receive, as these specialists order and perform more tests, more procedures, and more surgery. And they are the ones whose incomes will drop the most if they are placed on salary and no longer have the financial incentives to provide excessive services.

In addition to using "socialized medicine" and "government control of health care" as buzzwords to persuade the electorate and the politicians to reject comprehensive reform, organized medicine will probably also claim that the quality of care will suffer if cost constraints are instituted. Proponents of reform, however, will be able to show that the opposite is actually true, as confirmed by the outcomes in other developed nations. If unnecessary care is reduced and proper care is advanced, there will be less adverse events and quality will actually improve.

There are also large numbers of physicians who will be in favor of comprehensive reform and will support measures that control costs. Many of them want their patients to receive the best care, knowing that the system in place is not working and that monetary considerations are improperly influencing the way some of their colleagues practice. There is also the one-third of U.S. physicians who are already on salary and will have no objections to that payment option becoming universal. In addition, many primary care physicians will back comprehensive reform because it will offer them the possibility of increased remuneration, even as the income of some specialists is being reduced. It may even come to pass that major organizations serving primary care physicians will at some point promote comprehensive reform at the behest of their members.

(A survey of all physicians to determine their stances on comprehensive health care reform would be of interest to the medical community, the politicians who would be working on the measure, and the general public. This could be performed by a nonprofit agency or foundation, or by the government itself, perhaps through the Department of Health and Human Services. Obviously, physicians' self-interest would be a major factor in their positions, and even if a majority of them were against comprehensive reform, the legislation should be enacted, as it is critical to the future economic health of the nation and the viability of the health care system.)

### The Health Insurance Industry

The health insurance industry has more to lose than any of the other opponents if comprehensive health reform becomes the law of the land. Aside from the Tier 2 and Tier 3 policies, insurance companies would be able to function only in organizational and administrative capacities with fixed-service contracts. This role would not be nearly as lucrative as writing insurance with its risks and profits, and collecting the premiums from enrollees and employers. Those firms that remained in health care would be compelled to downsize and would no longer be as profitable as they had been in the past, working on contracts with strictly controlled payment schedules. It is possible, in fact, that some would be forced to go out of business. Certainly, the CEOs and other top executives would not be able to generate the kinds of benefit packages they had previously commanded, as the companies' income and growth would not warrant the same remuneration.

In addition to the cuts in executives' compensation, some would lose their jobs along with many lower level employees. The large administrative staffs of these companies would become superfluous, as there would be no more preapprovals for tests and procedures, or conflicts with physicians and patients over payments. Many of these laid-off employees would find positions with Universal Medicare or the RHEs, but some would have to look for work in other fields. Besides the impact on insurance company employees and executives, the stockholders of these companies would also be affected as the stocks declined in value. All of the people potentially harmed by the reform bill can be expected to actively oppose its passage, even though it would be a positive development for the majority of Americans. Thus, it can be anticipated that the health insurance companies and their lobbying machine, who brought the nation the "Harry and Louise" ads in the 1990s, would be working full blast to derail any attempts at comprehensive reform.

In their fight, the insurance companies would likely raise the same issues as organized medicine through their spokespeople on the radio and TV talk shows and in their advertisements. Comprehensive reform would be labeled as socialized medicine under government control, and they would bemoan the lower quality of care that would inevitably occur if the measure was enacted. They would also speak of Americans losing their freedom of choice under Universal Medicare, unable to make decisions about the type of coverage they wanted. Of course, very few Americans are able to select their own health insurance specifications under the current system. Their policies are usually chosen by their employers, or they are under the umbrella of Medicare or Medicaid. Those who are not covered either go without insurance or settle for low cost policies because it is all they can afford. If Universal Medicare were passed, people would still have the option of remaining outside the system and would also have the freedom to choose any of the Tier 2 plans, or Tier 3 coverages. There would actually be more freedom of choice for them, and affordability for basic care would no longer be a consideration.

The insurance companies and their surrogates would also likely emphasize the importance of market-based solutions to solve the problems of health care, saying that this is the American way. They would declare that Americans wouldn't want a program that delivered medical services utilizing some British concepts, or some Canadian ideas, or employed some French procedures (even though these countries have succeeded in providing universal coverage in a cost-effective manner). The insurance companies would also try to frighten people about the delays they would encounter in testing and treatment, which they would insist were bound to occur with the new program; having to wait weeks or months for an MRI or CT scan that would reveal whether there was cancer present, followed by long waits to have surgery to remove the lesion; or long waits to have a hip or knee replaced; or for coronary artery stenting, or bypass surgery. Of course, none of this would be true, since the same medical personnel would be in place who are there now, with the same imaging units and surgical suites. In fact, if unnecessary procedures and surgery were reduced or eliminated, physicians would be able to address real problems more expeditiously, and waiting times for tests and procedures would be decreased.

### The Pharmaceutical and Medical Device Industries

There would also be intense opposition to comprehensive reform from the pharmaceutical and medical device industries, with their concerns about both cost constraints and the negotiating power that would be granted to Universal Medicare. These industries are content with the current arrangements for buying and selling prescription drugs and medical devices and are strongly resistant to having them changed. With comprehensive reform, Universal Medicare would have great bargaining power over the prices of medical products, being the major buyer in the U.S. market. Thus, the drug companies would be forced to compete against each other in terms of price and effectiveness with any medications that were similar in function and mechanism. For instance, there are five or six statins (cholesterol-lowering drugs), including generics, all made by different pharmaceutical firms, which are comparable in the way they work. And there are a number of different prescription and over-the-counter proton-pump inhibitors that reduce acid production in the stomach and are used to treat ulcers and gastroesophageal reflux disease. Each drug company would try to have its product in these two classes become the preferred medication for Universal Medicare by touting its proficiency and lowering its price. This type of competition would take place across the board for every class of drug in the fight to have the preferred medications. Of course, other medications in each class would still be available, but would only be used if there were adverse reactions or failure of the preferred medications.

Under the current health care system, both traditional drug companies and generic manufacturers are thriving. If competitive bidding were introduced, new generic drug companies might also enter the fray, damaging the older generic companies by lowering prices for popular drugs even further. This extra competition might provide added help for Universal Medicare in its quest to control costs.

Some products are unique, with no competitors in their classes. This is particularly true of biopharmaceutical therapies that cost astronomical sums to treat various illnesses. Universal Medicare would negotiate with the firms that produce these compounds to try and obtain reasonable prices. However, if the negotiations were unsuccessful, UM might have to invoke cost/benefit ratios in deciding whether to continue using them, or to find alternative treatment options utilizing different substances that could work nearly as well. But the process and decision-making would be analytic and orderly, controlled by UM. This would be unlike the market for pharmaceuticals that exists today, where the drug companies have the upper hand and are free to raise prices as they desire. The drug companies would also be opposed to independent evaluation of their products, where benefits may be found to be overstated or nonexistent, or not as robust as those of competitors. Results of these evaluations could lead to a loss of income or to a product being dropped from Universal Medicare's formulary.

The medical device and equipment companies would also have to go the route of competitive bidding to have their products chosen by Universal Medicare. Those that are less costly and perform well in the tasks for which they are designed would be the ones preferred by UM. The era of having fixed prices being set by the device manufacturers and being paid by the government or insurance companies would be over.

The pharmaceutical and medical device industries would presumably employ some of the same arguments as organized medicine and the insurance companies in their attempts to mobilize the public and Congress against comprehensive reform. They would claim that quality would suffer and there would be no freedom of choice. They would assert that under the reform program, doctors might be unable to choose the devices or drugs they favored and might have to go with the low-cost options that Universal Medicare approved. They would further claim that this would compromise quality, as the preferred products would not necessarily be the best ones in their class. However, in actuality, Universal Medicare would be required to choose products of demonstrated effectiveness, in addition to considering price. And if a drug proved not to work or caused an adverse reaction, another medication would be substituted and covered by UM, even if it was not a primarily preferred product.

In addition, the drug and device companies and their advocates would likely claim (as they currently do) that their high prices were necessary to support the costs of research and compensate them for the expenses of generating new products. The companies would also say that if comprehensive reform allowed Universal Medicare to negotiate lower prices, innovation would suffer, with less money for research and development, and fewer new products available to bring to market. They would likely infer that cures for diseases such as cancer, multiple sclerosis, and Alzheimer's would be less apt to be discovered if reform was instituted, to the detriment of the public. In response, it should be asked why Americans should pay significantly more for their medications and devices than patients in other developed countries, and whether Americans alone should have to subsidize medical research (given the lower prices elsewhere). Government agencies currently are able to negotiate prices with the drug and device companies in these other countries. Why shouldn't Americans be able to get the same deals? Does free-market ideology require that Americans pay more for their medical products?

Medical research is also occurring in universities and federally supported laboratories across the nation, creating new drugs to address medicine's most urgent problems. Many of these products are licensed to pharmaceutical companies to be further tested and brought to market. The drug companies are not saddled by the research costs for these compounds, but they profit from manufacturing and selling them at lofty prices. Medical device companies benefit similarly when new products are developed with federal funding and are licensed by them. Under comprehensive reform, this pipeline would still remain open.

The new methods of purchasing medical products and the policies of cost constraint under Universal Medicare should not be fatal to the drug and device companies, but should rein in some of the excess gains, while still allowing them to remain quite profitable.

### The Hospitals

Many hospitals, both for-profit and nonprofit institutions, would be against reform because of its financial impact and the loss of local control. Hospitals might suffer financial privation if unnecessary services were reduced, as many of these procedures and operations generate funds for them. Determining care on the basis of cost/benefit ratios with a fixed annual budget for health care might also result in a drop in hospitals' income. The overriding of local control with centralized planning by Universal Medicare would be a major change in the climate for U.S. hospitals, with a stress on efficiency and a rational allocation of hospital beds. This would result in the closing of some institutions, decreasing the beds of some others, changing the missions and responsibilities of some hospitals, and regionalization of services in some areas. For all of these reasons, some hospital employees and executives would probably lose their jobs in the reorganization that occurred.

In addition, many communities that have economically precarious hospitals would pressure their legislative representatives to vote against comprehensive reform, fearful that their hospitals might be closed under the new program. Their residents would then have to travel further to obtain medical services and local unemployment might rise. Hospitals also contribute to the identities of some communities, and the emotional attachment to them is strong, making the possibility of closings even more distressing. National advertising campaigns might be undertaken by hospital associations to persuade voters and elected officials to oppose comprehensive reform, similar to those likely to be mounted by medical societies, the insurance, and pharmaceutical industries. In contrast, however, the hospitals would probably also concentrate on grass roots organizing to convince their congressmen, congresswomen, and senators to vote against the measure. In their opposition, local parochial interests would trump the greater common good that would be served by comprehensive reform.

### Trial Lawyers

The trial lawyers would be staunchly opposed to comprehensive reform, particularly the measures aimed at restructuring the malpractice process. With a more rational method of dealing with malpractice problems, plaintiffs' attorneys who handle these cases would likely see their incomes reduced. The American Association for Justice (formally the Trial Lawyers Association) would, therefore, undoubtedly fight reform aggressively, using lobbyists and advertisements to try and convince legislators and the public that grievously injured patients would not be adequately compensated if the bill were enacted. The arguments for malpractice reform, which include simplifying the system and using experts to determine malpractice, are straightforward and persuasive, and proponents should be able to refute any points that the trial lawyers put forth.

### The Unions

While the vast majority of U.S. unions would be strongly in favor of comprehensive reform, a number of them, whose members face possible job losses if the program was passed, would be opposed. These would include the unions that represent hospital workers, administrative employees of insurance companies, and workers in the pharmaceutical and medical device industries. Since most unions and their members throughout the country would be backing comprehensive reform, those against it would probably refrain from mounting national advertising campaigns attacking reform, but might hire their own lobbyists to challenge enactment. Grass roots pressure on elected officials to vote against reform might be used as well. Even as they acted to protect their own members, there would be a certain amount of ambivalence, knowing that comprehensive reform would be quite advantageous for other working men and women. These unions would also know that their brothers and sisters in the union movement would be fighting hard to counter their efforts, to ensure passage of the comprehensive reform bill.

### Alternative Health Practitioners

Alternative health practitioners, particularly chiropractors, would be united in opposition to comprehensive health care reform. With the cost constraints that are essential to the program and the requirement that treatments be of proven efficacy before they are reimbursed, these practitioners would not be eligible for payment by Universal Medicare. (Chiropractors may be compensated for some lower back care that has been shown to be beneficial.) Thus, they would try to mobilize patients, friends, and families in an attempt to block passage of the reform program, claiming that people were being denied freedom of choice in their care. Of course, people would not be prevented from using alternative practitioners, but would have to pay for the treatments themselves. Of all the alternative practitioners, chiropractors are the strongest numerically and politically. One can assume they would be working diligently to prevent comprehensive reform, using both grass roots organizations and national advertising campaigns.

## Confronting the Obstacles to Reform

As has been shown, the current health care system is not working, with runaway costs, failure to provide universal coverage, and inconsistent quality of care. Because of unconstrained spending on health care and the resulting obligations of Medicare and Medicaid, the nation has assumed trillions of dollars in unfunded liabilities, the burden of which will fall on the shoulders of succeeding generations. Health care costs have also damaged the competitiveness of U.S. businesses in the global economy and consumed funds that could have gone to education, research, defense, or national security. The principal proposals for reforming health care focus on providing coverage to those who are outside the system, but do not offer sound recommendations for controlling or lowering spending. Because of the lack of plausible measures to curb expenditures (among other flaws), none of the plans currently being advanced will be successful. If any of these incremental proposals are enacted, Congress will undoubtedly be searching again, within a short period of time, for new ways to tame the health care beast, and the country will suffer from yet another prolonged debate on the subject. A solution to the health care crisis, comprehensive reform, is staring politicians in the face. But they must be willing to break with the past and confront the powerful lobbyists and special interests arrayed against this program if they are to pass a bill that will bring relief to embattled U.S. consumers and businesses.

The obstacles to comprehensive health care reform are substantial, but they must be pushed aside. Though the evidence supporting the need for this legislation is overwhelming, the opposition will be brutal and unstinting as it battles against reform. Because of the effects of unconstrained health care costs on individual Americans and its destructive impact on the economy, the sooner legislation enabling reform is passed, the better it will be for the country. Realistically, however, the political climate must be right for such an extraordinary measure to be enacted. Perhaps now is the right time, given the recent financial upheavals, government intervention in the markets, and the additional pressures on the average U.S. family. But it is also possible that Americans will have to suffer even more pain before Congress has the will to take the great leap forward. If comprehensive health care reform is not passed in the current session of Congress, it will be at some point in the future. There is no reasonable alternative.

(Support for comprehensive health care reform could be mobilized through the Internet, as was successfully done to elect President Obama. This could counteract the advertising campaign against the bill by the lobbyists and special interests.)

Nothing is more dangerous than the influence of private interests in public affairs, and the abuse of the laws by the government is a less evil than the corruption of the legislator. . . . In such a case, the State being altered in substance, all reformation becomes impossible.

Jean-Jacques Rousseau[5]

# CHAPTER 9

# CONCLUSION

A long habit of not thinking a thing wrong, gives it a superficial appearance of being right.

—Thomas Paine, *Common Sense*[1]

The U.S. health care system is in dire straits, though the magnitude of its distress may not yet be apparent to all of its citizens who are aware only of the particular difficulties that affect them directly. These include the rising cost of health insurance; the increase in deductibles and co-pays that hit them in the pocketbook; the near impossibility of getting insurance if they have lost their jobs, are older, or have "preexisting conditions"; the denials for medical services or treatments by insurance companies who want to bolster their profits; and the nearly 46 million people without any coverage (undoubtedly much higher now with unemployment rising). These are some of the immediate problems plaguing the health care system that Americans live with every day.

However, in addition to these current concerns, the long-term trend of incessantly rising health care costs, over and beyond the rate of inflation, portends disaster for the economy and the country at some point in the future. The portion of the U.S. GDP devoted to health care has exploded from single digits two decades ago, to 16 percent today, with 20 percent predicted by 2016, and possibly 30 percent in the ensuing years. This translates to one in every five, or nearly one in every three dollars of the goods and services produced by the United States being in the realm of health care. The consequences of these statistics may be difficult to comprehend, but it means that health care spending will dwarf every other sector of the nation's economy, with less money available to spend in other critical areas. This is also unfair from a generational standpoint, since the bulk of health care expenditures are for older people and the money is taken from projects that would benefit all of the nation's citizens.

There is also the issue of the future unfunded liabilities of Medicare and Medicaid, which are estimated to be in the trillions to tens of trillions of dollars. This momentous problem has arisen due to the unchecked growth in health care costs, combined with the needs of an aging population, and is also unfair to younger Americans. The burden of this debt will fall upon the backs of today's children and their children if a way is not found to staunch the bleeding and constrain health care spending. This aspect of the health care crisis is not understood by the vast majority of Americans, nor has it been publicized by elected officials, who do not want to heighten anxiety among their constituents. And it has not been emphasized by the media, who perhaps do not find it a "sexy" enough story with high drama to engage their viewers or readers.

For anyone to argue that there currently is no health care crisis would indicate a disconnect from reality. The U.S. health care system is badly broken, and transformational change must be accomplished to prevent the cataclysm that will engulf the nation's economy if proper action is not taken. The programs now being proposed are prescriptions for failure and will require health care reform to be revisited at some time in the future. Albert Einstein once defined insanity as "doing the same thing over and over and expecting a different result." The United States has had minor health care reform measures enacted a number of times in the past without the desired results, and incremental, step-by-step, half measures that temporarily fill a pothole will not do the trick when a huge sinkhole is looming. Comprehensive health care reform, as detailed earlier, is the answer. To bring health care costs under control, administrative expenditures, unnecessary care, and fraud must all be dramatically curtailed, not withstanding the pain this will cause for the special interests in the health care industry.

The United States needs a single-payer system run by an independent entity, Universal Medicare, controlled by a board of health care experts, free of political interference. It must have a fixed budget and physicians must be paid by salary (as is now the case with about one-third of all doctors) to eliminate their incentives to increase services. (Entrepreneurial behavior by physicians within the scope of their medical practices must be ended.) Drug prices should be negotiated with the pharmaceutical companies, making certain that patients (and the health care system) get the best deals possible. Electronic health care records must be mandatory for every patient and the health care system must emphasize preventive care. With these measures enacted as part of comprehensive reform, enough savings can be generated to provide universal health care, bringing coverage to everyone without additional expenditures. General tax revenues should not have to be raised to fund this redesigned system. Financing it will simply require redirecting the money currently being spent in a more effective fashion to reduce waste and excessive care. Indeed, with realistic cost constraints in place, there is no reason the increase in health care spending could not be kept at (or even below) the rate of general inflation. Even more important, the specter of the system's unfunded liabilities would no longer hang over the heads of U.S. children like the sword of Damocles, waiting to destroy the dreams of tomorrow. (The cumulative savings under Universal Medicare could possibly surpass the money spent on the financial bailout.)

The new system, Universal Medicare, would not be government-controlled, but government-supported (and assisted in the collection of funds). It would not be "socialized medicine" because its structure would be entirely separate from the government, with health care managed by an independent board and regional entities. In fact, current government programs such as Medicare and Medicaid would be eliminated and absorbed into the new system, which would not be dependent on the much maligned government bureaucracy to function. Strict oversight would be instituted at multiple levels, with checks and balances to eliminate fraud and conflicts of interest. Personnel would be carefully monitored and would be accountable for their actions (the positive as well as the negative), and would be responsive to the people they serve, as well as to those issuing directives to them. And there would be no politics infecting the organism from the outside.

Though comprehensive reform would provide universal access to care, reduce costs, and bring the United States' unfunded liabilities to heel, what would it mean for patients on a daily basis? First of all, the new system would not interfere with doctor-patient relationships. Those that are already in place could be continued if so desired. Efforts would be made as well to increase the number of primary care physicians and physician extenders, to allow all Americans to receive optimum basic care. An emphasis on prevention would also mean healthier patients and less chronic diseases (which should also result in lower costs). There would not be long waits for tests or treatments, as sweeping the excess out of the system would free up time slots for required services. In addition, the marked reduction or elimination of unnecessary care would mean that patients weren't having unwarranted procedures or therapy with the adverse effects that can result. Measures to improve quality, malpractice reform, better oversight, and the use of electronic medical records would significantly decrease medical negligence as well, preserving lives, improving patient safety, and saving money. Better care would also produce better outcomes. Life expectancy should increase, infant mortality should drop, and quality of life should improve across the board. With the amount of money the United States currently spends on health care, there is no reason why it should be ranked near the bottom of developed nations on outcomes and standards of care parameters. With comprehensive reform established, the United States could aspire to be number one and could provide its citizens with the kind of care they deserve (and have paid for).

Many of the special interests in the health care industry will not be happy if comprehensive reform is enacted, but U.S. citizens will be the beneficiaries. Some of the features of the reform plan will also be opposed by politicians on both sides of the aisle, but there are tradeoffs that Republicans and Democrats can point to that will make the package more acceptable. Though conservatives may disagree with a single-payer system and the reduction of market forces in the health care system, they should favor malpractice reform and curbing the powers of litigation attorneys. Liberals may find the change in malpractice procedures unpalatable, but they should be satisfied with the other aspects of comprehensive reform. Hopefully, both Republicans and Democrats will be able to work together to ensure that the empowering legislation includes all the components of the program.

Using a budget to control costs raises the question of whether rationing of care might become necessary if budgetary limits were exceeded. In all likelihood this would never come to pass, as the cost savings built into the program will be substantial. However, cost/benefit ratios will be used to determine whether procedures or services are worthwhile, and ineffective treatments or unproductive tests will not be eligible for reimbursement. Certainly, this is better than the system now being utilized, where rationing regularly occurs as determined by the quality of a person's health insurance or what he or she can afford out-of-pocket.

Given the seismic changes that have recently roiled the financial system, with the federal government bailing out and buying into the banks, the unprecedented rescue of a major insurance company, and the loans offered to the auto companies, there is an opening now for a major restructuring of the health care system. Established concepts regarding the workings of the economy have been shattered, and ideas that were previously anathema to Americans are now being accepted by most citizens because they have been deemed necessary to rescue floundering institutions. Similar innovation is needed to rescue the failing U.S. health care system. Moreover, the current economic turmoil and projected federal deficits over the next several years should not be used as reasons to delay or derail comprehensive reform. Universal Medicare will not require funding beyond what is already being spent on health care and, in fact, could contribute savings to help meet the nation's budgetary demands. In the 1930s, during the Great Depression, Social Security was passed when the economy was at its nadir. Health care reform now is as critical as Social Security was then, particularly with the spike in unemployment and the additional millions of Americans without health insurance. There is a great opportunity at hand to control a burgeoning crisis. Hopefully, it will not be missed.

However, the difficulty President Obama had shortly after assuming the presidency in passing the economic stimulus bill without bipartisan support, foreshadows the problems that can be expected in trying to enact comprehensive health care reform. To overcome the threat of a Republican filibuster and garner a few extra votes, the Democrats had to make major compromises in the legislation, eliminating or reducing some of the Obama administration's requests. If the Republicans, with a handful of conservative Democrats, choose to back the insurance companies and insist that there are viable market-based solutions to the health care crisis, comprehensive reform will be unable to pass in this session of Congress. Perhaps, then, in the elections to follow, health care reform can be used as a lever to assemble a filibuster-proof majority on this issue, and comprehensive reform can finally become a reality.

# NOTES

## Chapter 1

1. Jean-Jacques Rousseau, *The Social Contract*, E. P. Dutton, New York, 1950, p. 102. Originally published in French, in 1762.

2. Tom Daschle, *Critical—What We Can Do about the Health Care Crisis?* St Martin's Press, New York, 2008, p. 53.

3. Vincente Navarro, "Federal Health Policies in the United States: An Alternative Explanation," in *The Nation's Health*, 3rd Edition, edited by Philip Lee and Carroll Estes Jones, Bartlett, Boston, 1990, p. 160.

4. Steven A. Schroeder, "We Can Do Better—Improving the Health of the American People," *New England Journal of Medicine* 2007; 357:1221–1228.

5. Stephen Ohlemacher, "US Lags behind 41 Nations in Life Span," AOL News, 8/13/07.

6. Reed Abelson, "While the U.S. Spends Heavily on Health Care, a Study Faults the Quality," *New York Times*, July 17, 2008, p. C3.

7. Ohlemacher, op cit.

8. Doug Trapp, "Uninsured Tally Dips to 45.7 Million with More Covered by Government," *American Medical News*, September 15, 2008, 51(35):1

9. Chris L. Peterson and Rachael Burton, "U.S. Health Care Spending: Comparison with Other OECD Countries," *CRS Report to Congress*, September 17, 2007, http://assets.opencrs.com/rpts/RL34175_20070917.pdf.

10. "Maybe I'll Get Better on My Own," Editorial, *New York Times*, June 30, 2008, p. A18.

11. Douglas Waller, "How VA Hospitals Became the Best," *Time*, September 4, 2006, p. 36.

12. Robert Pear, "Bush Seeks Surplus via Medicare Cuts," *New York Times*, January 31, 2008, p. A18.

13. "Medicare's Much-Too-Hard Sell," Editorial, *New York Times*, May 21, 2008, p. A28.

14. Robert Pear, "For Recipients of Medicare, the Hard Sell," *New York Times*, December 17, 2007, p. A1.

15. Ezekiel J. Emanuel and Victor R. Fuchs, "The Perfect Storm of Overutilization," *JAMA* 2008; 299:1789–1791.

16. Ibid.

17. Shannon Brownlee, "The Overtreated American," in *The Real State of the Union*, New American Library, New York, 2004, p. 130.

18. Ibid., p. 132.

19. John E. Wennberg, Elliott S. Fisher, and Jonathan Skinner, "Geography and the Debate over Medicare Reform," *Health Affairs*, Web Exclusive, 2002, W96–114.

20. "Facts on Health Care Costs," National Coalition on Health Care, 2006, http://www.nchc.org/facts/cost.shtml.

21. "Health Care for Automakers: A Progressive Priority for America," Center for American Progress, http://www.americanprogress.org/issues/2006/11/auto_industry .html.

22. Ezekiel J. Emanuel and Victor R. Fuchs, "Who Really Pays for Health Care?" *JAMA* 2008; 299:1057–1059.

23. Doug Trapp, "Health Outlay Tops $2 Trillion, but Spending Growth on Doctors Declines," *American Medical News*, January 28, 2008, p. 1.

24. Julie Appleby, "Health Spending Rises at Blistering Pace," *USA Today*, June 9, 2006, p. B1.

25. Gina Kolata, "Making Health Care the Engine That Drives the Economy," *New York Times*, August 22, 2006, p. F5.

26. "Facts on Health Care Costs," 2006.

27. Julie Appleby, June 9, 2006.

28. Ibid.

29. Robert Pear, "Outlook Remains Bleak for 2 Programs," *New York Times*, March 26, 2008, p. A15.

30. David A. Wells, Joseph S. Ross, and Allan S. Detsky, "What Is Different about the Market for Health Care?" *JAMA* 2007; 298:2785–2787.

31. "Rating Your Doctor, Fairly," Editorial, *New York Times*, December 8, 2007, p. A26.

32. Pamela Lewis Dolan, "Patients Rarely Use Online Ratings to Pick Physicians," *American Medical News*, June 23/30, 2008, p. 1.

33. Steffie Woolhandler and David Himmelstein, "When Money Is the Mission—The High Costs of Investor-Owned Care," *New England Journal of Medicine* 1999; 341:444–446.

34. Ibid.

35. Daniel Gross, "National Health Care? We're Halfway There," Economic View, *New York Times*, December 3, 2006, Business 4.

36. David Cay Johnston, "Competitively Priced Electricity Costs More, Studies Show," *New York Times*, November 6, 2007, p. C4.

37. Paul Krugman, "Voodoo Health Economics," *New York Times*, Op-Ed, April 4, 2008, p. A23.

## Chapter 2

1. David Hume, *Enquiries Concerning Human Understanding*, 3rd Edition, Oxford University Press, New York, 1975, p. 87 (reprinted from the posthumous edition of 1777).

2. Roy Porter, *The Greatest Benefit to Mankind*, W.W. Norton, New York, 1997, p. 289.

3. "A Brief History of Osteopathy," www.cranialacademy.com/history.html.

4. "History of Chiropractic Medicine," http://wikipedia.org/wiki/chiropractic_history.

5. "Germ Theory of Disease," http://en.wikipedia.org/wiki/Germ_theory_of_disease.

6. Isaac M. McPhee, "The History of Anesthesia," February 3, 2008, http://generalmedicine.suite101.com/article.cfm/the_history_of_anesthesia.

7. "Surgery," http://en.wikipedia.org/wiki/Surgery.

8. "William Halstead," http://en.wikipedia.org/wiki/William_Halstead.

9. J. T. H. Connor, "The Victorian Revolution in Surgery," *Science*, April 2, 2004, 304(5667):54–55.

10. "History of the American Society of Radiologic Technologists," www.asrt.org/content/aboutasrt/history.aspx.

11. Molly Cooke et al., "American Medical Education 100 Years after the Flexner Report," *New England Journal of Medicine* 2006; 355:1339–1344.

12. Donald Melnick et al., "Medical Licensing Examinations in the United States," *Journal of Dental Education* 2002; 66:595–599.

13. "Kaiser Permanente," http://en.wikipedia.org/wiki/Kaiser_Permanente.

14. Darrell G. Kirch and David J. Vernon, "Confronting the Complexity of the Physician Workforce Equation," *JAMA* 2008; 299:2680–2682.

15. Ibid.

16. Ibid.

17. Sandeep Jauhar, "Eyes Bloodshot, Doctors Vent Their Discontent," *New York Times*, June 17, 2008, p. F5.

18. Doug Trapp, "Law Prohibits Employer and Insurer Genetic Discrimination," *American Medical News*, June 6, 2008, p. 5.

19. James P. Evans, "Health Care in the Age of Genetic Medicine," *JAMA* 2007; 298:2670–2672.

20. "The Health Insurance Portability and Accountability Act," http://en.wikipedia.org/wiki/HIPAA.

21. "Our Pen-and-Pencil Doctors," Editorial, *New York Times*, June 24, 2008, p. A22.

22. Letter to Physicians from Health Net (Insurance Company), May 29, 2008, CSMS IPA.

23. Steve Lohr, "Microsoft Offers System to Track Health Records," *International Herald Tribune*, October 5, 2007, p. 13.

24. David Glendinning, "E-prescribers See Medicare Bonus, but Late Adopters Will Face Pay Cut," *American Medical News*, August 4, 2008, p. 1.

25. Paul Starr, *The Social Transformation of American Medicine*, Basic Books, New York, 1982, pp. 88–90.

26. Frederick E. Sondern, "Brief History of Organized Medicine," *Bulletin of the New York Academy of Medicine* 1936; 12(1):1–13.

27. Ibid.

28. Starr, op. cit., p. 99.

29. Ibid., p. 109.

30. Ibid., p. 92.

31. Ibid., p. 110.

32. "American Medical Association," *United States History Encyclopedia*, www.answers.com/topic/american-medical-association?cat=health.

33. "National Health Insurance," *Encyclopedia of Public Health*, www.enotes.com/public-health-encyclopedia/national-health-insurance/.

34. "American Medical Association," op. cit.

35. "American Medical Association," http://en.wikipedia.org/wiki/American_Medical _Association.

36. "National Health Insurance," op. cit.

37. David Blumenthal, "Health Care Reform—Past and Future," *New England Journal of Medicine* 1995; 332:465–468.

38. Jonathan Oberlander, "The Politics of Medicare Reform," *Washington and Lee Law Review*, Fall 2003.

39. John K. Iglehart, "Medicare's Declining Payments to Physicians," *New England Journal of Medicine* 2002; 346:1924–1930.

40. Robert Pear, "Congress, Overriding Bus, Blocks Pay Cut for Doctors," *New York Times*, July 16, 2008, p. A13.

41. Robert Pear, "Long-Term Fix Is Elusive in Medicare Payments," *New York Times*, July 13, 2008, p. 18.

42. Laura B. Powers, "MEM: Working to Help Keep Neurologists in Practice," *AANnews*, November 2007, p. 3.

43. Stephanie Maxwell et al., "Use of Physicians' Services under Medicare's Resource-Based Payments," *New England Journal of Medicine* 2007; 356:1853–1861.

44. Oberlander, op. cit.

45. Peter P. Budetti, "Market Justice and US Health Care," *JAMA* 2008; 299:92–94.

46. "National Health Insurance," op cit.

47. Oberlander, op. cit.

48. Robert E. Moffit, "The Success of Medicare Advantage Plans: What Seniors Should Know," Executive Summary Backgrounder, The Heritage Foundation, No. 2142, June 13, 2008.

49. "Medicare's Bias," Editorial, *New York Times*, July 14, 2008, p. A16.

50. Moffit, op. cit.

51. Dana P. Goldman and Geoffrey F. Joyce, "Medicare Part D—A Successful Start with Room for Improvement," *JAMA* 2008; 299:1954–1955.

52. Ibid.

53. David Boddiger, "AMA hopes streamlined agenda will boost membership," *The Lancet* 2005; 366:971–972.

## Chapter 3

1. David Hume, *Enquiries Concerning Human Understanding and Concerning the Principles of Morals*, Clarendon Press, Oxford Press, New York, 1994, p. 47 (originally published in 1748 and 1751).

2. Paul Starr, *The Social Transformation of American Medicine*, Basic Books, New York, 1982, pp. 145, 147, 148.

3. Anthony Kovner, "Hospitals," in *Health Care Delivery in the United States*, Springer Publishing Company, New York, 1990, pp. 141–174.

4. Jennie Jacobs Kronenfeld, *Health Care Policy—Issue and Trends*, Greenwood Publishing, Westport, CT, pp. 65–79.

5. A. Assaf et al., "Possible Influence of the Prospective Payment System on the Assignment of Discharge Diagnoses for Coronary Heart Disease," *New England Journal of Medicine* 1993; 317:867.

6. Kronenfeld, op. cit.

7. Ibid.

8. "Physicians and Surgeons," U.S. Department of Labor, Bureau of Labor Statistics, December 18, 2007, http://www.bls.gov/oco/ocos074.htm.

9. Janice Hopkins Tanne, "Mortality Higher at For-Profit Hospitals," *BMJ* 2002; 324:1351.

10. Steffie Woolhandler and David U. Himmelstein, "When Money Is the Mission— The High Costs of Investor-Owned Care," *New England Journal of Medicine* 1999; 341:444–446.

11. Ibid.

12. Janice Hopkins Tanne, op. cit.

13. Ibid.

14. Elaine M. Silverman et al., "The Association between For-Profit Hospital Ownership and Increased Medicare Spending," *New England Journal of Medicine* 1999; 341:420–426.

15. P. J. Deveraux et al., "Payments for Care at Private For-Profit and Private Not-for-Profit Hospitals: A Systemic Review and Meta-Analysis," *Canadian Medical Association Journal*, June 8, 2004, pp. 1817–1824.

16. Steffie Woolhandler and David U. Himmelstein, "The High Costs of For-Profit Care," *Canadian Medical Association Journal*, June 8, 2004, pp. 1814–1815.

17. Elaine Silverman and Jonathan Skinner, "Are For-Profit Hospitals Really Different? Medicare Upcoding and Market Structure," *IDEAS*, 6/18/08, http://ideas.repec .org/p/nbr/nberwo/8133.html.

18. Pushkal P. Garg et al., "Effect of the Ownership of Dialysis Facilities on Patients' Survival and Referral for Transplantation," *New England Journal of Medicine* 1999; 341:1653–1660.

19. "Specialty Hospitals," GAO Report to Congressional Requesters, October 2003, www.gao.gov/new.items/d04167.pdf.

20. Ibid.

21. Robert Pear, "Concerned about Costs, Congress Pushes Curbs on Doctor-Owned Hospitals," *New York Times*, June 8, 2008, p. 22.

22. Melissa Thomasson, "Health Insurance in the United States," *EH.Net Encyclopedia*, http://eh.net/encyclopedia/article/thomasson.insurance.health.us.

23. Ibid.

24. David Blumenthal, "Employer-Sponsored Health Insurance in the United States— Origins and Implications," *New England Journal of Medicine* 2006; 355:82–88.

25. Ibid.

26. Thomasson, op. cit.

27. Blumenthal, op. cit.

28. Ibid.

29. "Managed Care," *Encyclopedia of Public Health*, Answers.com, www.answers.com/ topic/managed-care?cat=biz-fin.

30. "A Brief History of Managed Care," Tufts Managed Care Institute, http://63.251 .142.241/downloads/BriefHist.pdf.

31. Ibid.

32. Starr, op. cit., p. 396.

33. "A Brief History of Managed Care," op. cit.

34. "Managed Care," op. cit.

35. Reed Abelson, "Small Business Is Latest Focus in Health Care Fight," *New York Times*, July 10, 2008, p. A1.

36. "Lowering Medicare Drug Prices," Editorial, *New York Times*, November 26, 2006, p. A26.

37. "FDA Public Health Advisory: Safety of Vioxx," September 30, 2004, http://www.fda.gov/CDER/Drug/infopage/vioxx/PHA_vioxx.htm.

38. Rita Rubin, "How Did Vioxx Debacle Happen?" *USA Today*, October 12, 2004, p. A1.

39. "Vioxx May Have Caused 140,000 Heart Attacks," www.consumeraffairs.com/news04/2005/vioxx_lancet.html.

40. Alice Park, "Is Vytorin a Failure?" *Time*, January 15, 2008, www.time.com/time/printout/0,8816,1703827,00.html.

41. Ezekiel J. Emanuel and Victor R. Fuchs, "The Perfect Storm of Overutilization," *JAMA* 2008; 299:2789–2791.

42. Ashley Wazana, "Physicians and the Pharmaceutical Industry," *JAMA* 2000; 283:373–380.

43. Myrle Croasdale, "Med Schools Asked to Shun Drug Firm Freebies," *American Medical News*, May 26, 2008, p. 1.

44. Kevin B. O'Reilly, "Drug Industry: No More Free Pens, Pads, or Mugs," *American Medical News*, July 28, 2008, p. 1.

45. Gardiner Harris and Benedict Carey, "Researchers Fail to Reveal Full Drug Pay," *New York Times*, June 8, 2008, p. A1.

46. Stephanie Saul, "Drug Ads Raise Questions for Heart Pioneer," *New York Times*, February 7, 2008, p. A1.

47. Julie M. Donohue et al., "A Decade of Direct-to-Consumer Advertising of Prescription Drugs," *New England Journal of Medicine* 2007; 357:673–681.

48. Stephanie Saul and Alex Berenson, "Maker of Lipitor Digs In to Fight Generic Rival," *New York Times*, November 3, 2007, p. 1.

49. Ibid.

50. "Unsafe Medical Devices Remain Serious Problem," Consumers Union, 2007, http://www.consumersunion.org/pub/core_health_care/004484.html.

51. Ibid.

52. David Leonhardt, "High Medicare Costs, Courtesy of Congress," *New York Times*, June 25, 2008, p. C1.

### Chapter 4

1. Franz Kafka, *The Castle*, Vintage Books, Alfred A. Knopf, New York, 1974, p. 333. Originally published in German in 1930.

2. Robert Pear, "Gap in Life Expectancy Widens for the Nation," *New York Times*, March 23, 2008, p. 19.

3. J. Michael Williams et al., "Health of Previously Uninsured Adults after Acquiring Medicare Coverage," *JAMA* 2007; 298:2886–2894.

4. "Illnesses and Medical Bills Cause Half of All Bankruptcies," New Release, Harvard Medical School Office of Public Affairs, February 2, 2005, http://hms.harvard.edu/public/news/relsum2005.html.

5. Robert Pear, "Bush Seeks Surplus via Medicare Cuts," *New York Times*, January 21, 2008, p. A18.

6. "How Changes in Medical Technology Affect Health Care Costs," *Snapshots: Health Care Costs*, The Henry J. Kaiser Foundation, March 2007, http://www.kff.org/insurance/snapshot/chcm030807oth.cfm.

7. S. Burner et al., "Nation's Health Care Expenditures Projections through 2030," *Health Care Financing Review* 1992; 14(1):4.

8. Donald D. Hensrud and Samuel Klein, "Extreme Obesity: A New Medical Crisis in the United States," *Mayo Clinic Proceedings* 2006; 81(10suppl):S5–S10.

9. Donald D. Hensrud and M. Molly McMahon, "Bariatric Surgery in Adults With Extreme (Not Morbid) Obesity," *Mayo Clinic Proceedings* 2006; 81(10suppl):S3–S4.

10. Hensrud and Klein, op. cit.

11. Jane Brody, "Panel Urges Hour of Exercise a Day; Sets Diet Guidelines," *New York Times*, September 6, 2002, www.NYTimes.com.

12. Smoking 101 Fact Sheet, American Lung Association, http://www.lungusa.org/site/c.dvLUK9O0E/b.39853/k.5D05/Smoking_101_Fact_Sheet.htm.

13. Ibid.

14. http://www.cdc.gov/tobacco/data_statistics/fact_sheets/adult_data/adult_cig_smoking.htm.

15. "The Economic Costs of Drug Abuse in the United States, 1992–2002," www.whitehousedrugpolicy.gov/publications/economic_costs/.

16. "Alcohol Alert #51, National Institute on Alcohol Abuse and Alcoholism," January 2001, http://pubs.niaaa.nih.gov/publications/aa51.htm.

17. *Snapshots*, The Henry J. Kaiser Foundation, op. cit.

18. Ibid.

19. Ibid.

20. "The Growth in Diagnostic Imaging Utilization" (Pennsylvania Hospital Commission), www.phc4.org/reports/fyi/fyi27.htm.

21. Ibid.

22. http://www.petscaninfo.com/zportal/portals/pat/faq.

23. "Trend: Growth in CT Scans Concerns Some," January 15, 2008, www.fiercehealthcare.com/story/trend-growth-ct-scans-concerns-some/2008-01-15.

24. "The Growth in Diagnostic Imaging Utilization," op. cit.

25. Alex Berenson and Reed Abelson, "Weighing the Costs of a CT Scan's Look inside the Heart," *New York Times*, June 29, 2008, p. A1.

26. Rita F. Redberg and Judith Walsh, "Pay Now, Benefits May Follow—The Case of Cardiac Computed Tomographic Angiography," *New England Journal of Medicine* 2008; 359:2309–2311.

27. Ibid.

28. Andrew Pollack, "Hospitals Look to Nuclear Tool to Fight Cancer," *New York Times*, December 7, 2007, p. A1.

29. Matthew Herper, "Losing Lipitor," 7/18/07, http://www.forbes.com/2007/07/18/pharmaceuticals-pfizer-lipitor-biz-sci-cx_mh_0718pfizer.html.

30. Julie Appleby, "More Using Prescription Drugs," *USA Today*, February 13, 2008, p. 1A.

31. "Cerezyme," www.drugs.com/cdi/cerezyme.html.

32. Andrew Pollack, "Cutting Dosage of Costly Drug Spurs a Debate," *New York Times*, March 16, 2007, www.NYTimes.com.

33. "Bevacizumab Combined with Chemotherapy Prolongs Survival for Some Patients with Advanced Lung Cancer," *National Cancer Institute News*, 5/13/05, http://www.cancer.gov/newscenter/pressreleases/AvastinLung.

34. Andrew Pollack, "F.D.A. Extends Avastin's Use to Breast Cancer," *New York Times*, February 23, 2008, p. C1.

35. Gina Kolata and Andre Pollack, "Costly Cancer Drug Offers Hope, but Also a Dilemma," *New York Times*, July 6, 2008, p. 1.

36. Robert Steinbeck, "The Price of Sight-Ranizumab, Bevacizumab, and the Treatment of Macular Degeneration," *New England Journal of Medicine* 2006; 355: 1409–1412.

37. Reed Abelson and Andrew Pollack, "Medicare Widens Drugs It Accepts for Cancer," *New York Times*, January 27, 2009, p. A1.

38. Louise M. Slaughter, "Medicare Part D—The Product of a Broken Process," *New England Journal of Medicine* 2006; 354:2314–2315.

39. Ibid.

40. Alex Berenson, "Big Drug Makers Post Profits That Beat Forecasts," *New York Times*, July 25, 2006, p. C1.

41. Milt Freudenheim, "Drug Prices Up Sharply This Year," *New York Times*, June 21, 2006, p. C1.

42. Julie Appleby, "Health Spending Rises at Blistering Pace," *USA Today*, June 9, 2006, p. B1.

43. Chris L. Peterson and Rachael Burton, "U.S. Health Care Spending: Comparison with Other O.E.C.D. Countries," CRS Report to Congress, September 17, 2007, http://assets.opencrs.com/rpts/RL34175_20070917.pdf.

44. Ibid.

45. Ibid.

46. Saritha Rai, "Union Disrupts Plan to Send Ailing Workers to India for Cheaper Medical Care," *New York Times*, October 11, 2006, p. C6.

47. Barnaby J. Feder, "A Heart Stent Maker Decides the Way to the Patient Is through the Patient," *New York Times*, December 5, 2007, p. C3.

48. Barry Meier, "Consumer Ads for Medical Devices Subject of Senate Panel," *New York Times*, September 15, 2008, p. C1

49. Thomas Goetz, "Practicing Patients," *New York Times Sunday Magazine*, March 23, 2008, p. 32.

50. Barron H. Lerner, "Choosing a 'God Squad,' When the Mind Has Faded," *New York Times*, August 29, 2006, p. F5.

51. Ibid.

52. Julie Appleby, "End of Life Costs," *USA Today*, October 19, 2006, p. 1A.

53. Robert Pear, "Researchers Find Huge Variations in End-of-Life Treatment," *New York Times*, April 7, 2008, p. A17.

54. Ibid.

55. Anemona Hartocollis, "Rise Seen in Medical Efforts to Improve Very Long Lives," *New York Times*, July 18, 2008, p. A1.

56. Roger Reynolds et al., "The Cost of Medical Professional Liability," *JAMA* 1987; 257:2776–2781.

57. John Carroll, "Going on the Offensive Against Defensive Medicine," Managed Care, March 2005, http://www.managedcaremag.com/archives/0503/0503.regulation.html.

58. David U. Himmelstein, Steffie Woolhandler, and Sidney Wolfe, "Administrative Waste in the U.S. Health Care System in 2003," *International Journal of Health Services* 2004; 34(1):79–86.

59. Eric Alterman and George Zornick, "Think Again: An Unhealthy Dialogue on Health Care," Center for American Progress Action Fund, February 7, 2008, http://www.americanprogressaction.org/issues/2008/unhealthy_dialogue.html.

60. Tyler Cowen, "Abolishing the Middleman Won't Make Health Care a Free Lunch," *New York Times*, Business, March 22, 2007, www.NYTimes.com.

61. Ibid.

62. "Healthcare Fraud," UnitedHealthcare Oxford, March 2008, https://www.oxhp .com/main/fraud.html.

63. "Healthcare Fraud and You," BlueCross, BlueShield, March 2008, http://www .fepblue.org/about/fraud.html.

64. "Fraud," Department of Health and Human Services and the Department of Justice, Health Care Fraud and Abuse Control Program, Annual Report for FY 2000, January 2001.

65. "Largest Health Care Fraud Case in U.S. History Settled," Department of Justice, June 26, 2003, http://www.integriguard.org/corp/newsevents/pressreleases/2003/ 2003-06-26.html.

66. Evelyn Pringle, "Gambro Healthcare—Dialysis Fraud Pays Big Bucks," April 3, 2006, http://www.scoop.co.nz/stories/HL0604/S00007.htm.

67. Robert Pear, "Report Links Dead Doctors to Payments by Medicare," *New York Times*, July 9, 2008, p. A16.

68. David Glendinning, "Medicare Audit Overreach?" *American Medical News*, July 7, 2008, p. 5.

69. John E. Wennberg, Elliot S. Fisher, and Jonathan Skinner, "Geography and the Debate Over Medicare Reform," *Health Affairs*, Web Exclusive, 2002, W96–W114.

70. Shannon Brownlee, "The Overtreated American," in *The Real State of the Union*, edited by Ted Halstead, Basic Books, New York, 2004.

71. Peter R Orzag, "Opportunities to Increase Efficiency in Health Care," Congressional Budget Office, June 16, 2008.

72. "Are Most Hysterectomies Unnecessary?" *ABC News*, August 27, 2004, http:// abcnews.go.com/print?id=124229.

73. The Associated Press, "Study: Most Angioplasties Unnecessary," March, 26, 2007, MSNBC, www.msnbc.msn.com/id/17800298/print/1/displaymode/1098/.

74. William E. Boden et al., "Optimal Medical Therapy with or without PCI for Stable Coronary Disease," *New England Journal of Medicine* 2007; 356:1503–1516.

75. G. R. Tait et al., "Unnecessary Arthroscopies," *Injury* 1992; 23:555–556.

76. J. Weinstein et al., "Surgical Versus Nonoperative Treatment for Lumbar Disk Herniation," *JAMA* 2006; 296:2441–2450.

77. Richard A. Deyo et al., "Spinal Fusion: The Case for Restraint," *New England Journal of Medicine* 2004; 350:722–726.

78. Ibid.

79. Leslie Berger, "Back Pain Eludes Perfect Solutions" *New York Times*, May 13, 2008, Wellness Section, p. 8.

80. Richard A. Deyo, op. cit.

81. Alex Berenson and Andrew Pollack, "Doctors Reap Millions for Anemia Drugs," *New York Times*, May 7, 2007, p. A1.

82. Jeanne Linzer, "Health care group agrees $500 million settlement for unnecessary surgery," *BMJ* 2006; 333(7558):59.

83. Milt Freudenheim, "Trying to Save by Increasing Doctors' Fees," *New York Times*, May 21, 2007, p. A1.

84. Michael Arnold Glueck and Robert J. Cihak, "High Cost of Care for Illegal Immigrants," December 27, 2005, newsmax.com, http://archive.newsmax.com/archives/ articles/2005/12/26/170334.shtml.

85. George Anders, "UnitedHealth Directors Strive to Please Chief," *The Wall Street Journal*, April 18, 2006, http://www.post-gazette.com/pg/06108/68305428.stm.

86. Ibid.

87. "How Can a $124 Million a Year CEO Make Health Care More Affordable?" *Health Care Renewal*, May 10, 2005, http://hcrenewal.blogspot.com/2005/05/how-can-1248-million-year-ceo-make.html.

88. Emily Berry, "Health Plans Say They'll Risk Losing Members to Protect Profit Margins," *American Medical News*, May 19, 2008, p. 1.

89. Ibid.

90. Kurt Samson, "UnitedHealth Charged with Data Manipulation Scheme," *Neurology Today* 2008; 8(6):1.

91. Gina Kolata, "Co-Payments Soar for Drugs with High Prices," *New York Times*, April 14, 2008, p. A1.

92. Mary Ellen Schneider, "New Drug Pricing Structure Angers Patients, Doctors," *Clinical Neurology News* 2008; 4(5):1.

93. Kevin Sack, "Study Finds Cancer Diagnosis Linked to Insurance," *New York Times*, February 18, 2008, p. A10.

94. Doug Trapp, "Health Care Access Problems Surge among Insured Americans," *American Medical News*, July 21, 2008, p. 1.

95. "Coalition to Advance Health Care Reform," www.coalition4healthcare.org/.

96. Ibid., Ronald A. Williams, Chairman, CEO and President, Aetna.

97. Robert Steinbrook, "Medical Student Debt—Is There a Limit?" *New England Journal of Medicine* 2008; 359:2629–2632.

98. Wayne J. Guglielmo, "Physician Earnings: Our Exclusive Survey," *Medical Economics*, September 19, 2003.

99. "U.S. Physician Salaries Ongoing Salary Survey," www.allied-physicians.com/salary_surveys/physician-salaries.htm.

100. "Physicians Group Predicts Family Doctor Shortages in at Least Five States by 2020," *Medical News Today*, September 29, 2006, http://www.medicalnewstoday.com/articles/52884.php.

101. James Arvantes, "Primary Care Physician Shortage Creates Medically Disenfranchised Population, aafp news now, Washington, D.C., 3/22/2007, ttp://www.aafp.org/online/en/home/publications/news/news-now/professionalissues/20070322disenfranchised.html.

102. Nancy Shute, "Can't Find a Doctor? You're Not Alone," *U.S. News and World Report*, March 19, 2008, http://health.usnews.com/articles/health/living-well-usn/2008/03/19/cant-find-a-doctor-youre-not-alone.html.

103. Myrle Croasdale, "Shortage of General Surgeons Is Straining Some Facilities," *American Medical News*, June 2, 2008, p. 10.

104. Ibid.

105. Louis Uchitelle, "Lure of Great Wealth Affects Career Choices," *New York Times*, November 27, 2006, p. A1.

106. Natasha Singer, "For Top Medical Students, an Attractive Field," *New York Times*, March 19, 2008, p. A1.

107. Natasha Singer, "As Doctors Cater to Looks, Skin Patients Wait," *New York Times*, July 28, 2008, p. A1.

## Chapter 5

1. Robert Wachter and Kaveh Shojania, *Internal Bleeding—The Truth Behind America's Terrifying Epidemic of Medical Mistakes*, Rugged Land, New York, 2004, p. 297.

2. Philip K. Howard, *The Death Of Common Sense.* Random House, New York, 1994, p. 23 (quoting Justice Benjamin Cardozo).

3. James C. Mohr, "American Medical Malpractice Litigation in Historical Perspective," *JAMA* 2000; 283:1731.

4. Andrew H. Smith, "Medical Error and Patient Injury: Costly and Often Preventable," AARP Public Policy Institute, September 1998, http://www.aarp.org/research/health/carequality/aresearch-import-711-IB35.html.

5. Donald M. Berwick and Lucian L. Leape, "Reducing Errors in Medicine," Editorial, *BMJ* 1999; 319:136–137.

6. T. A. Brennan et al., "Incidence of Adverse Events and Negligence in Hospitalized Patients: Results of the Harvard Practice Study," *New England Journal of Medicine* 1991; 324:370–376.

7. Berwick and Leape, op. cit.

8. Richard Anderson, "An 'Epidemic' of Medical Malpractice? A Commentary on the Harvard Medical Practice Study," Civil Justice Memo No. 27, July 1996, Manhattan Institute for Policy Research, www.manhattan-institute.org/html/cjm_27.htm.

9. Ibid.

10. "To Err Is Human: Building a Safer Health Care System," *Institute of Medicine,* November 1999, p. 1.

11. Christopher J. Conover, "Medical Tort System," Center for Health Policy, Law and Management, Duke University, May 2004, http://www.hpolicy.duke.edu/cyberexchange/Regulate/CHSR/HTMLs/MTS1-MedicalTortSystem.htm.

12. Lucian L. Leape and Donald M. Berwick, "Five Years after *To Err Is Human*—What Have We Learned?" *JAMA* 2005; 293:2384–2390.

13. Robert Pear, "Medicare Says It Won't Cover Hospital Errors," *New York Times,* August 19, 2007, p. A1.

14. Peter J. Pronovost et al., "The Wisdom and Justice of Not Paying for 'Preventable Complications,'" *JAMA* 2008; 299:2197–2199.

15. Roger Reynolds, John Rizzo, and Martin Gonzalez. "The Cost of Medical Professional Liability." *JAMA* 1987; 257:2776–2781.

16. Christopher J. Conover, op. cit.

17. Zac Haughn, "Examining the Health of Medical Malpractice Coverage," *Practical Neurology,* April 2008, p. 16–23.

18. Ibid.

19. Wyatt Andrews, "Defensive Medicine: Cautious or Costly?" CBS News, October 22, 2007, www.cbsnews.com/stories/2007/10/22/eveingnews/printable3394654.shtml.

20. Christopher J. Conover, op. cit.

21. "Confronting the New Health Care Crisis: Improving Health Care Quality and Lowering Costs by Fixing Our Medical Liability System," Department of Health and Human Services, July 24, 2002, http://aspe.hhs.gov/daltcp/reports/litrefm.pdf.

22. Ibid.

23. Ibid.

24. Helen Burstin et al., *JAMA* 1993; 270:1697–1701.

25. Troyen Brennan et al., "Relation Between Negligent Adverse Events and the Outcomes of Medical Malpractice Litigation," *New England Journal of Medicine* 1996; 335:1963–1967.

26. "Confronting the Health Care Crisis," op. cit.

27. Ibid.

28. Ibid.

29. Hubert Winston Smith, "Legal Responsibility For Medical Malpractice," *JAMA* 1941; 116:942.

30. "National Practitioner Data Bank," *AMA Legal Issues,* National Practitioner Data Bank, February 5, 2008, www.ama-assn.org/ama/pub/category/4543.html.

31. LaRae Huycke and Mark Huycke, "Characteristics of Potential Plaintiffs in Malpractice Litigation," *Annals of Internal Medicine* 1994; 120:792–798.

32. Howard Beckman et al., "The Doctor-Patient Relationship and Malpractice," *Archives of Internal Medicine* 1994; 154:1365–1370.

33. Thomas H. Gallagher et al., "Disclosing Harmful Medical Errors to Patients," *New England Journal of Medicine* 2007; 356:2713–2719.

34. Adam Liptak, "In U.S., Expert Witnesses Are Partisan," *New York Times,* August 12, 2008, p. A1.

35. Philip K. Howard, *The Death Of Common Sense,* Random House, New York, 1994, p. 44.

36. Walter K. Olson, *The Rule of Lawyers,* St Martin's Press, New York, 2003, pp. 265–266.

## Chapter 6

1. Marcus Aurelius, *Meditations,* Walter J. Black, Inc., Roslyn, NY, 1945, p. 40.

2. Cathy Schoen et al., "Bending the Curve: Options for Achieving Savings and Improving Value in U.S. Health Care Spending," *The Commonwealth Fund,* December 18, 2007, Vol. 80, http://www.cmwf.org/Content/Publications/Fund-Reports/2007/Dec/Bending-the-Curve—Options-for-Achieving-Savings-and-Improving-Value-in-U-S—Health-Spending.aspx.

3. Doug Trapp, "Latest Medicare Projections Renew Alarm on Long-Term Sustainability," *American Medical News,* April 14, 2008, p. 1.

4. "The High Cost of Health Care," Editorial, *New York Times,* November 25, 2007, Week in Review, p. 9.

5. Laurence J. Kotlikoff, *The Healthcare Fix,* The MIT Press, Cambridge, MA, 2007, pp. 3–7.

6. Stephen M. Shortell and Lawrence P. Casalino, "Health Care Reform Requires Accountable Care Systems," *JAMA* 2008; 300:95–97.

7. "Most Docs Want Health System Reform," *American Medical News,* May 19, 2008, p. 7.

8. Jonathan Oberlander, "The Politics of Medicare Reform," *Washington and Lee Law Review,* Fall 2003, http://findarticles.com/p/articles/mi_qa3655/is_200310/ai_n9262300.

9. Kotlikoff, op. cit., p. 22.

10. Steffie Woolhandler and David U. Himmelstein, "When Money Is the Mission—The High Costs of Investor-Owned Care," *New England Journal of Medicine* 1999; 341:444–446.

11. W. A. Glaser, "The United States Needs a Health System Like Other Countries," *JAMA* 1993; 270:980–984.

12. Jim McDermott, "Evaluating Health System Reform: The Case for a Single-Payer Approach," *JAMA* 1994; 782–784.

13. David U. Himmelstein and Steffie Woolhandler, "I Am Not a Health Reform," *New York Times,* Op-Ed, December 15, 2007, p. A23.

14. Tyler Cowen, "Abolishing the Middleman Won't Make Health Care a Free Lunch," *New York Times*, May 22, 2007, p. C3.

15. Tom Daschle, Jeanne Lambrew, and Scott Greenberger, *Critical*, Thomas Dunne Books, New York, 2008, p. 169–180.

16. Robert Pear, "Fed Chief Addresses Health Care and Its Costs," *New York Times*, June 17, 2008, p. A15.

17. John M. Eisenberg, "Ten Lessons for Evidence-Based Technology Assessment," *JAMA* 1999; 282:1865–1872.

18. Seymour Perry and Mae Thamer, "Medical Innovation and the Critical Role of HealthTechnology Assessment," *JAMA* 1999; 282:1869–1872.

19. Gardiner Harris, "British Balance Benefit vs. Cost of Latest Drugs," *New York Times*, December 3, 2008, p. A1.

20. Schoen, op cit.

21. Robert Pear, "Senate Bars Medicare Talks for Lower Prices on Drugs," *New York Times*, April 19, 2007, p. A20.

22. Schoen, op. cit.

23. James F. Fries et al., "Reducing Health Care Costs by Reducing the Need and Demand for Medical Services," *New England Journal of Medicine* 1993; 329:321–324.

24. Ibid.

25. Schoen, op. cit.

26. "Single-Payer FAQ," Physicians for a National Health Program, www.pnhp.org/facts/singlepayer_faq.php.

27. Pamela Villarreal, "Federal Medicaid Funding Reform," National Center for Policy Analysis, July 31, 2006, www.ncpa.org/pub/ba/ba566/.

28. R. H. Brook et al., "Does Free Care Improve Adults' Health? Results from a Randomized Controlled Trial," *New England Journal of Medicine* 1983; 309:1426–1434.

29. David A. Wells et al., "What Is Different about the Market for Health Care?" *JAMA* 2007; 298:2785–2787.

30. "Single-Payer FAQ," op. cit.

31. Gerard F. Anderson and Kalipso Chalkidou, "Spending on Medical Care—More Is Better?" *JAMA* 2008; 299:2444–2445.

32. Floyd J. Fowler Jr. et al., "Relationship between Regional Per Capita Medicare Expenditures and Patient Perceptions of Quality of Care," *JAMA* 2008; 299:2406–2412.

33. Shannon Brownlee, "Overdose," *The Atlantic*, December 2007, p. 36–38.

34. Kotlikoff, op. cit., p. 17–18.

35. Deborah Epstein, "Keeping Salaried Physicians Satisfied and Productive," *Managed Care Magazine*, March 1996, www.managedcaremag.com/archives/9603/MC9603 .salaried.shtml.

36. Ibid.

37. Ibid.

38. Karen E. Hauer et al., "Factors Associated With Medical Students' Career Choices Regarding Internal Medicine," *JAMA* 2008; 300:1154–1164.

39. David C. Goodman, "Improving Accountability for the Public Investment in Health Profession Education," *JAMA* 2008; 300:1205–1207.

40. Meredith B. Rosenthal, "Beyond Pay for Performance—Emerging Models of Provider-Payment Reform," *New England Journal of Medicine* 2008; 359:1197–1200.

41. John K. Iglehart, "No Place Like Home—Testing a New Model of Care Delivery," *New England Journal of Medicine* 2008; 359:1200–1202.

42. Elliot S. Fisher, "Building a Medical Neighborhood for the Medical Home," *New England Journal of Medicine* 2008; 359:1202–1205.

43. Myrie Croasdale, "Harvard Offers Discount on Med School Tuition," *American Medical News*, May 12, 2008, p. 12.

44. Emily Berry, "Who's behind the Card?" *American Medical News*, August 25, 2008, p. 11.

45. Timothy Stolzfus Jost and Ezekiel J. Emmanuel, "Legal Reforms Necessary to Promote Delivery System Innovation," *JAMA* 2008; 299:2561–2563.

46. "E-Prescribing Overview," Centers for Medicare and Medicaid Services, 4/15/2008, www.cms.hhs.gov/eprescribing/.

47. Dave Hansen, "Deadline Does Not Compute," *American Medical News*, May 19, 2008, p. 9–10.

48. Christine Larson, "Yes, the P.A. Will See You Now," *New York Times*, Business, August 10, 2008, p. 10.

49. Mary O. Mundinger et al., "Primary Care Outcomes in Patients Treated by Nurse Practitioners or Physicians," *JAMA* 2000; 283:59–68.

50. Fries et al., op. cit.

51. Myrle Croasdale, "Advanced-practice Nurses Seek Wider Scope in 24 States," *American Medical News*, April 21, 2008, p. 1.

## Chapter 7

1. Thomas Paine, *Common Sense*, Penguin Books, New York, 1986, p. 68 (originally published in 1776).

2. Jonathan Cohn, "What's the One Thing Big Business and the Left Have in Common?" *New York Times*, April 1, 2007, www.NYTimes.com.

3. Senator John McCain, "Access to Quality and Affordable Health Care for Every American," *New England Journal of Medicine* 2008; 359:1537–1541.

4. Senator Barack Obama, "Modern Health Care for All Americans," *New England Journal of Medicine* 2008; 359:1537–1541.

5. Jonel Aleccia, "Overhauling Health Care: Two Divergent Visions," MSNBC.com, September 22, 2008, http://www.msnbc.msn.com/id/26761504/.

6. Jonathan Oberlander, "The Partisan Divide—The McCain and Obama Plans for U.S. Health Care Reform," *New England Journal of Medicine* 2008; 359:781–784.

7. Ibid.

8. Editorial, "McCain vs Obama on Health Care," *The Lancet* 2008; 371:1971.

9. Doug Trapp, "Sept. 1, 2008. Campaign Case Report: What Obama and McCain Pledge to Do about the Health System," (Government), *American Medical News* 2008; 51:5.

10. Thomas Buchmueller et al., "Cost and Coverage Implications of the McCain Plan to Restructure Health Insurance," *Health Affairs* 2008; 27:472–481.

11. Aleccia, op. cit.

12. David Blumenthal, "Primum Non Nocere—The McCain Plan for Health Insecurity," *New England Journal of Medicine* 2008; 359:1645–1647.

13. Buchmueller, op. cit.

14. Ibid.

15. Kevin Sack, "McCain Plan to Aid States on Health Could Be Costly," *New York Times*, July 8, 2008, p. A1.

16. Kevin Sack, "Business Cool Toward McCain's Health Coverage Plan," *New York Times*, October 7, 2008, p. A20.

17. Oberlander, op. cit.

18. Ibid.

19. Joseph Antos, Gail Wilensky, and Hanns Kuttner, "The Obama Plan: More Regulation, Unsustainable Spending," *Health Affairs* 2008; 27:462–471.

20. Obama, op. cit.

21. Editorial, *The Lancet*, op. cit.

22. Kevin Sack, "Health Plan From Obama Spurs Debate," *New York Times*, July 23, 2008, p. A1.

23. Trapp, op. cit.

24. Obama, op. cit.

25. Antos, Wilensky, and Kuttner, op. cit.

26. Oberlander, op. cit.

27. Eric Berger, "McCain and Obama on Emergency Care: The Candidates' Approach to Emergency Care," *Annals of Emergency Medicine* 2008; 52:265–267.

28. Stephen Morrissey, Gregory Curfman, and Jeffrey M. Drazen, "Health of the Nation—Coverage for All Americans," *New England Journal of Medicine* 2008; 359:855–856.

29. Antos, Wilensky, and Kuttner, op. cit.

30. Ibid.

31. Joseph R. Antos, "Symptomatic Relief, but No Cure—The Obama Health Care Reform," *New England Journal of Medicine* 2008; 359:1648–1650.

32. H. Gilbert Welch, "Campaign Myth: Prevention as Cure-All," *New York Times*, October 7, 2008, p. D6.

33. Stuart H. Altman and Michael Doonan, "Can Massachusetts Lead the Way in Health Care Reform?" *New England Journal of Medicine* 2006; 354:2093–2095.

34. Robert Steinbrook, "Health Care Reform in Massachusetts—A Work in Progress," *New England Journal of Medicine* 2006; 354:2095–2098.

35. Editorial, "The Massachusetts Way," *New York Times*, August 30, 2008, p. A18.

36. Kevin Sack, "Study Finds State Gains in Insurance," *New York Times*, June 3, 2008, p. A14.

37. Doug Trapp, "Are Mandates Ready For Prime Time?" *American Medical News*, June 2, 2008, p. 5.

38. Kevin Sack, "New Florida Law Allows Low-Cost Health Policies," *New York Times*, May 22, 2008, p. A22.

39. Kevin Sack, "Health Care Issue, Not Quite Hot, Remains Strong," *New York Times*, September 12, 2008, p. A20.

40. Milt Freudenheim, "Mayo Clinic Recommends Universal Health Insurance Plan," *New York Times*, September 15, 2008, p. B4.

41. Ashley Smith, "AMA-endorsed Health-care Plan Focuses on Choice," *New Hampshire Business Review*, January 18, 2008, http://www.allbusiness.com/insurance/health-insurance-government-health-national/6781530-1.html.

42. "Response to AMA's Health Care Reform Proposal," American Student Medical Association, June 17, 2008, www.amsa.org/uhc/response_AMA.cfm.

43. "The NHS—Organisation and Structure," Economics of Health Care, www.oheschools.org/ohech4pg2.html.

44. "The Structure of the NHS," November, 2004, www.rcgp.org.uk/pdf/ISS_info_08_Nov04.pdf.

45. Stephen Campbell et al., "Quality of Primary Care in England with the Introduction of Pay for Performance," *New England Journal of Medicine* 2007; 357:181–190.

46. "The Structure of the NHS," op. cit.

47. "The NHS—Organisation and Structure," op. cit.

48. "UK National Health Service," Answers.com, 10/9/2008, www.answers.com/topic/national-health-service.

49. Ibid.

50. Ibid.

51. Sarah Lyall, "Paying Patients Test British Health System," *New York Times*, February 21, 2008, p. A12.

52. "Medicare (Canada), Wikipedia, 10/9/08, www.en.wikipedia.org/wiki/Medicare_(Canada).

53. "Single-Payer FAQ," Physicians for a National Health Program," 4/25/2008, www.pnhp.org/facts/singlepayer_faq.php.

54. "Health Care in Germany," National Coalition on Health Care," 10/18/08, http://www.nchc.org/documents/Germany.pdf.

55. Ibid.

56. "Health Care in Germany," MedHunters.com 10/14/2008, www.medhunters.com/articles/healthcareInGermany.html.

57. Ibid.

58. "Health Care in Germany," National Coalition on Health Care, op. cit.

59. Ibid.

60. Ibid.

61. "Health Care in Germany," Medhunter, op. cit.

62. "Health Care in Germany," National Coalition on Health Care, op. cit.

63. Kerry Capell, "The French Lesson in Health Care," *BusinessWeek*, July 9, 2007, www.businessweek.com/print/magazine/content/07_28/b4042070.htm?chan=gl.

64. Mary Cline, "The Health Care System I Want Is in France," *ABC News*, April 15, 2008, http://abcnews.go.com/print?id=4647483.

65. Kerry Capell, op. cit.

66. Ibid.

67. "The French Health Care System," *Medical News Today*, June 27, 2004, www.medicalnewstoday.com/printerfriendlynews.php?newsid=9994.

68. Ibid.

69. Ibid.

70. Ibid.

71. Kerry Capell, op. cit.

72. *Medical News Today*, op. cit.

73. Joseph Shapiro, "Health Care Lessons from France," NPR, July 11, 2008, http://www.npr.org/templates/story/story.php?storyId=92419273.

74. T. R. Reid, "Japanese Pay Less for More Health Care," NPR, April 9, 2008, http://www.npr.org/templates/story/story.php?storyId=89626309.

75. "Health Care in Japan," National Coalition on Health Care," http://www.nchc.org/documents/Japan.pdf Obtained 10/26/08.

76. Johanna Ward & Cynthia M Piccolo, "Health Care in Japan," Medhunters.com, 10/26/08, http://www.medhunters.com/articles/healthcareInJapan.html.

77. T. R. Reid, op. cit.

78. Ward & Piccolo, op. cit.

79. Ibid.

80. "Health Care in Japan," National Coalition on Health Care, op. cit.

## Chapter 8

1. James Madison, *The Federalist Papers*, Number 62, New American Library, New York, 1961, p. 380 (originally appeared, 1787–1788).

2. Robert Pear, "Long-Term Fix Is Elusive in Medicare Payments, "*New York Times*, July 13, 2008, p. 18.

3. David Leonhardt, "High Medicare Costs, Courtesy of Congress," *New York Times*, June 25, 2008, p. C1.

4. Robert Steinbrook, "Election 2008—Campaign Contributions, Lobbying and the U.S. Health Sector," *New England Journal of Medicine* 2008; 357:736–739.

5. Jean-Jacques Rousseau, "The Social Contract and Discourses," E.P. Dutton and Company, New York, 1950, p. 65 (originally published in French in 1762).

## Chapter 9

1. Thomas Paine, *Common Sense*, Penguin Books, New York, 1986, p. 63 (originally published in 1776).

# INDEX

# ABOUT THE AUTHOR

ROBERT A. LEVINE, M.D., is a graduate of Columbia College and the Downstate Medical Center in Brooklyn. Dr. Levine served in Vietnam in the Army Medical Corps, then trained in neurology at the Albert Einstein Medical Center in the Bronx. Subsequently, he has been in private practice (neurology) in Norwalk, Connecticut. He is the former chief of neurology at Norwalk Hospital and an associate clinical professor of medicine at Yale University (ret.). He has published two previous books, *Aging with Attitude* and *Defying Dementia*. Since college, he has had a particular interest in politics and the delivery of health care.